Nursing Care of the Skin

Commissioning editor: Mary Seager
Development editor: Caroline Savage
Production controller: Anthony Read
Desk editor: Jackie Holding
Cover designer: Fred Rose

2013
DF

Nursing Care of the Skin

Edited by

Rebecca Penzer
BSc (Hons), PG Dip Adv. Prac., PG Dip Prof. Educ.

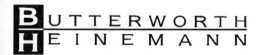
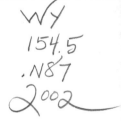

WY
154.5
.N87
2002

BUTTERWORTH
HEINEMANN

OXFORD   AUCKLAND   BOSTON   JOHANNESBURG   MELBOURNE   NEW DELHI

Butterworth-Heinemann
An imprint of Elsevier Science

First published 2002

British Library Cataloguing in Publication Data
Penzer, Rebecca
  Nursing care of the skin
  1. Dermatologic nursing   2.   Skin
  I. Title
  610.7'36

ISBN 0 7506 2834 0

Typeset by Keyword Typesetting Services Ltd, UK
Printed and bound in Great Britain by Biddles Ltd, Guildford and
King's Lynn

Contents

List of Contributors

Polly Buchanan BSc(Hons), RGN, RM, ONC, DipN
Consultant Nurse in Dermatology and Honorary Senior
Lecturer, Institute of Health Care Studies, Bournemouth
University, Bournemouth

Su Bullus RGN, DipN, RSCN, FETC
Dermatology Liaison Nurse, Dermatology Department, The
Churchill Hospital, Oxford Radcliffe NHS Trust, Oxford

Rebecca Davis BSc(Hons), RGN
Whipps Cross University Hospital NHS Trust, Leytonstone,
London

Rebecca Penzer RGN, BSc(Hons), PG Dip Adv. Prac., PG Dip
Prof. Educ.
International Project Co-ordinator, School of Nursing and
Midwifery, University of Southampton, Southampton

Fiona Pringle RGN FETC, ENB901
Clinical Nurse Manager, Oxford Fertility Unit Women's Centre,
Oxford Radcliffe NHS Trust, Oxford

Preface

During 5 years as a dermatology nurse I have become increasingly aware of the dearth of literature about caring for the skin. As a novice to dermatology I could not find a comprehensive nursing-oriented text that provided answers to my everyday questions. As I gained experience in the field it became clear to me that I was not alone. Nurses in other specialities as well as my own were hungry for skin-care knowledge, but were not able to find the information they required to inform their practice. This, therefore, is the aim of this text; to provide nurses from all specialities with skin-care information that will encourage and enable holistic, well-informed practice.

Skin problems are often chronic in nature. Chronic illness means that it is a longstanding problem for which there is no permanent cure. There may be periods of remission when overt signs and symptoms are not present, but the possibility of a relapse is ever present. Therefore the nurse's responsibility, as with all chronic illness, is not based on cure but instead on care. Any patient requiring care in any healthcare setting may have a chronic skin condition. Sensitive assessment of individual needs should be carried out to determine the precise areas where nursing care is needed, be it a physical or psychological intervention. Those people who do not have a chronic skin condition but an acute one, such as a drug reaction, will need intervention of a different kind. This care will not involve such extensive long-term planning or the development of coping strategies, but will nevertheless need great sensitivity.

Being able to provide quality skin care is essential in all fields of nursing. There are the obvious issues, such as preventing pressure sores and managing wound care, but alongside these commonly recognized areas of care are a myriad of other considerations. For patients to be able to carry out activities of living they require skin that functions correctly. Sore feet make walking impossible, cracked and painful hands make grooming, dressing and washing uncomfortable and often impossible, and of course being facially disfigured by acne makes social contacts embarrassing and may lead to isolation. Nurses must therefore have the knowledge and skills to tackle these physical and psychosocial difficulties. They will frequently exist alongside the primary reason for an individual coming into contact with healthcare professionals, either in the community or in hospitals, and within the context of holistic care must not be ignored.

The above shows that this book can and should be relevant for all nurses. All the contributors have avoided using the word 'dermatology', as we wanted to make the information as accessible as possible to the maximum number of nurses. It is primarily a practical book, and although theory is used to inform practice statements, the key focus is on action. To encourage further thought on topics, reflection points are given. The intention of these points is not only to encourage individual thought but also to give food for discussion with colleagues and/or ideas on particular areas that may benefit from further work.

Although chapters are written by individuals, there are some common themes running through them. These include the importance of age, culture/race, and privacy and dignity.

This book can be used as a complete text, and reading from cover to cover will provide sequential information. However, as already stated, the aim of this book is that it should be practical, and therefore dipping in and out of relevant bits should be easy using the index and subheadings within the text.

The book takes a humanistic/holistic approach towards skin care, the focus being on the care of patient problems rather than discussion of disease processes. This means that whilst disease names are included, what is of prime importance are the symptoms, how these affect patients and what nurses can do about them.

Chapter 1 kicks off by looking at how the skin can be assessed, and also how it can be used as an assessment tool to gain information about other disease processes that might be going on in the body. Ways of describing the skin are discussed, and terminology and jargon is unravelled so that you will no longer need to call every skin blemish 'a rash'.

Chapter 2 moves on to look at the structure and function of normal skin as well as how it should be cared for. The emphasis here is on health rather than disease. A variety of preventative strategies are highlighted, making this a very practical guide to skin care.

Chapter 3 complements the second chapter by looking at the skills needed to care for skin that is not functioning normally.

As mentioned previously, symptoms are the focus, although brief explanations of disease processes and altered physiology are made. Care is illuminated using case studies. A very broad range of topics is tackled, and these are supported with references to further information as needed.

Chapter 4 is a key chapter in that the discussion of body image brings up issues that must be considered when caring for anybody with compromised skin function. Whilst cursory mention is often made regarding the effects of skin disease on body image, this chapter is unique in the way that it brings together many generic issues and relates them to the effects of altered skin function.

Chapter 5 gives specific consideration to the needs of patients who have chronic skin conditions that they need help looking after when they are at home. This chapter gives special weight to common treatments in the community, alternative therapies, and patient support groups.

Chapter 6 concludes the book by discussing health education. Once again, generic theories and techniques are made relevant for those who need to teach people about caring for their skin.

This book is intended to be the start of your quest for knowledge about skin care. Even if it has answered all your current questions, I hope you will read the references so you can gain deeper knowledge of the subject. However you use this book, my main hope is that you feel empowered to make your patients more comfortable both physically and psychologically.

Rebecca Penzer

Planning care for someone with altered skin function

Rebecca Penzer

Introduction

Planning care for someone that has altered skin function is in many ways no different from planning care for someone with any other health problems. Consequently, although the aim of this chapter is to highlight ways in which care planning may be enhanced for those with skin problems, it will include many strategies that are useful when planning care for anyone. The first part of this chapter gives guidance about planning care through the use of the nursing process, and the second part of the chapter highlights some key themes that are important to underpin all the care offered to those with altered skin function.

Planning care requires rigorous assessment, logical, well-evidenced planning, and timely, caring intervention. Continual evaluation and reassessment must occur throughout the whole process. The use of the nursing process is key to ensuring this; however, several other strategies may be employed to ensure that accurate information is gathered and used. These strategies are laid out in this chapter in such a way that they can be used alongside any nursing model that is currently in use within the healthcare setting. Likewise they are sufficiently flexible for use within any environment, whether a hospital, a patient's home or a community practice. To clarify how all the various different strategies discussed fit together they have been summarized in Table 1.1. Each nursing process in the table will then be discussed in further detail.

No specific nursing model is recommended in this chapter, as the information gathered will need to be used within the model currently in use within the clinical area. Suffice it to say that a model is a useful way of guiding thinking about the processes required for planning care and thus focusing attention on particular areas of need – whether Orem's self-care model (Orem, 1985) or Roy's model of role identification (Roy, 1988). The intention of the following sections is to help nurses to make best use of

Table 1.1 Strategies for gathering information regarding skin problems

Specific strategies useful for attention to skin problems	Nursing process	Overall strategies for good practice
Using four of the five senses for assessment	Assessment	Use a nursing model or equivalent
Accurate descriptions of the lesions as they are seen	Problem identification (goal setting)	Use an open interview technique to gain information from the patient
Take a systems approach to guide assessment	Planning care	Document all information with care and without using judgemental statements
Use knowledge gained in this book	Implementation	Follow the UKCC's guidelines for record keeping
Using four of the five senses	Evaluation	Use a SOAP format for ongoing planning and evaluation of care

nursing models and the nursing process in the planning of care for patients with skin problems.

Before working through the nursing process, your attention is drawn to two key areas that need consideration; first, skills of interviewing, and second, those of accurate and useful documentation.

Interview techniques

Whichever model is in use, it is vital that its use does not restrict the assessment process to an interview based upon a rigid set of predetermined questions, which is followed without thought. Thinking of the initial assessment as a guided interview is helpful; what is key is that relevant information is gained in a way that makes patients feel confident in the care that they will receive. During an assessment, interview data that refer to objective and subjective perspectives of a patient's experience must be gained. Developing the skills required to carry out such an interview will take time. Using a model to guide the process is recommended, as it will provide reminders of vital areas that need to be covered.

Doenges and Moorhouse (1992) recommend 10 points that help to ensure a successful interview:

   1. *Underlying purpose.* Be clear what your purpose is. Usually the information gathered will be used to design the care plan, but

obviously these pointers for a good interview technique could be used in other situations – for example, interviewing a patient as part of a research project.

2. *Preliminary research.* Gather as much information prior to the interview as possible. This may come from nursing or medical notes. Try and identify key points that you want to investigate further.

3. *Request to conduct the interview.* This is a simple gesture that shows consideration of your patient as an individual, and respect for his or her privacy.

4. *Interview strategy.* Explain to the patient the purpose and general outline of the interview process. This just lets the patient know what to expect – for example, 'I'd like to ask you some questions about how you normally manage at home and how your symptoms have affected your life. Once we have done this, I will take your temperature, pulse and blood pressure'.

5. *Icebreakers.* These can be used at the start of the interview to put the patient at ease, perhaps by making a social comment or offering a drink. An icebreaker question can be helpful for collecting information; for example, 'How did you get here today?' or 'Who was that with you when you first arrived?' may give you some information about the patient's social set-up.

6. *Business.* Get to the business of the interview using your pre-planned strategy. Useful techniques to use include:

   - Open-ended questions that require more than a 'yes' or 'no' answer – e.g. 'Tell me how your skin makes you feel', rather than 'Does your skin make you feel bad?'
   - Hypothetical questions, which are 'what if?' questions – e.g. 'What if your skin were to suddenly start itching – what would you do?'
   - Reflecting or mirroring the responses obtained from the patient – e.g. the patient may say 'Sometimes I just feel like ignoring all my treatments, they take so long to do', and a reflective response to this could be 'Do you feel frustrated by all the treatments you have to do?'
   - Focusing, which involves getting the patient to go into more detail about a specific issue – e.g. the interviewer could ask the patient to 'Tell me more about all the treatments you need to do'. This can be accentuated by body language, such as leaning forward and maintaining an open posture.

7. *Rapport.* The best interviews will be achieved when a positive rapport is established with the patient. It is important not to

bore or intimidate the patient by using unfamiliar language and/or imposing body language. A positive rapport is most likely to be established if the other elements of the interview techniques highlighted above are adhered to – i.e. showing courtesy by asking for the interview to take place, indicating social skills by using icebreakers, and showing interest by the way you ask open questions.

8. *Sensitivity.* This is needed particularly with regard to potentially embarrassing questions. Questions regarding such issues of sexuality should not be ignored, as they are often of particular importance for those with skin disease. It may be that the initial interview is not the time to address them; however, their impact on the individual needs to be acknowledged.

9. *Recovery.* If a sensitive area is touched upon and it is clear that the patient does not feel comfortable in sharing the information, recovery needs to occur to allow the interview to continue in a useful and open manner. This will be more likely to occur when a good rapport has been established originally and by showing warmth through a smile or touch, for example.

10. *Closure.* End by summarizing the information that you have gained and asking if it is accurate. It is also important to allow an opportunity for the patient to add anything further or ask more questions.

The environment in which the interview is carried out is an important consideration. Finding somewhere that is soundproof is often difficult, if not impossible; however, somewhere that is relatively quiet and where the likelihood of interruption is kept to a minimum is ideal. If there is going to be the need to examine someone's skin, it is particularly important that an intrusion will not happen.

Documentation

Once the information has been gathered, it needs to be documented. Again, strategies for documentation will vary enormously; however, some overriding principles must be adhered to. United Kingdom Central Council (UKCC) guidelines on record keeping should be referred to for details. Whilst clearly any documentation must be legible and with a minimum of abbreviations, it should go further and be comprehensible to patients.

All documents should be written in such a way that minimizes the use of subjective statements. Subjective statements can refer to one or more of three themes:

1. *Time*. Words like 'often', 'sometimes' and 'rarely' all have little meaning in reality. They need to be much more specific; for example, refer to the number of times per day (e.g. three times per day).
2. *Quantities*. These should be specifically defined in terms of volume, weight, width etc. Saying 'some', 'a lot' or 'many' has little meaning and is subject to interpretation.
3. *Qualitative*. Subjective qualitative statements may be offensive as well as inaccurate. For example, referring to a 'demanding' or 'incompetent' patient involves making a judgement that is likely to have negative connotations. Thus the word not only fails to measure accurately just how demanding 'demanding' is – calling once a night or 10 times a night? – but it may also be derogatory. Objective statements, which describe how it is known that someone is as they are described in the notes, are vital. For example: 'Mr Bridges is very irritable today' is a subjective statement, whereas 'Mr Bridges said he felt particularly itchy today and expressed discontent with the fact that his treatment was delayed' is an objective statement. Although they take longer to write, objective statements give much more information about the patient and why they are feeling as they do, and are thus much more useful in terms of planning and evaluating care.

Nursing process

Assessment

The initial interview as described above is when much assessment takes place. However, assessment is an ongoing process and should not be thought of as a one-off event. Through the interview process it will become clear to what extent the skin problem impacts on the patient. If, for example, the patient has liver failure, jaundiced skin will be a product of this medical condition. Although this will have a psychological effect on the patient, which will need sensitive care, the physical care of the skin will revolve around resolving the medical problem – i.e. the patient's skin will remain yellow unless the liver failure is managed. However, on assessment of other patients you may become aware that the skin itself poses a major health problem for the individual – for example, there may be an actual or potential break in skin integrity, a chronic wound, an allergy or a skin disease.

Once it becomes clear that the skin is having an impact on the well-being of the patient, it is helpful to use a systems approach to assess how the problem affects that individual. The approach recommended here first considers the functions of the skin and then assesses whether the problems the patient is experiencing impact on this function.

Assessing function

The examples of questions below are by no means comprehensive. However, if the skin does appear to be functioning abnormally, taking a look at its various functions can give an indication of how the problem impacts on the individual.

Protection
The skin provides protection from the outside world; it is a barrier that keeps water, chemicals, foreign bodies and bacteria out and holds vital organs in. Therefore if the patient has a break in skin integrity or if there is a possibility that the skin might become broken, the following should be considered.

1. Are there any breaks in the skin?
2. What has caused these breaks?
3. Is there an infection?
4. Does the skin look vulnerable in any way?
5. Is the skin dry, blistered, thinning, easily bruised or itchy?

Psychosocial
There are two key things that can be established about a person when considering the psychosocial impact of a skin problem:

1. How the skin appears to the outside world and how people react to this
2. How the person copes with the way that he or she looks.

It may be that you notice how other people shy away from physical contact with the patient because of the way he or she looks, and you need to be aware of your own feelings and whether you feel like avoiding contact. This lack of contact may lead to social isolation for the patient, which is difficult at any time, but perhaps even harder to endure at times of ill health. Patients will themselves react in a very individual manner; they may seem unbothered, or they may choose to isolate themselves even if those around them are not averse to social contact.

Sensory

The sensory function is closely linked with protection, as it is the sensory nerve endings in the skin that allow us to move away from potential danger. There are two key questions to bear in mind:

1. Is there decreased sensation, as there might be in a patient with diabetic neuropathy?
2. Is there heightened sensation, as there may be in the skin surrounding a painful leg ulcer?

Storage

The skin is responsible for storing the body's supply of both fat and water, and therefore provides a very good way of assessing how well nourished and/or hydrated the patient is. Consider:

1. Is the patient malnourished, with a body mass index lower than average?
2. Is the patient at risk of developing pressure sores because there is no fatty protection?
3. Is the patient dehydrated? Does the skin look dry and when it is pinched up? Does it return to its usual shape or remain pinched up (a classic sign of dehydration)?

Absorption

The skin can absorb a number of substances; however, excessive absorption of ultraviolet light and/or certain chemicals can be damaging. Consider the following questions:

1. Ultraviolet light:
   - Is the patient sunburnt?
   - Are there any unusual moles that are itching or bleeding or that have increased in size recently?
   - Is the patient a sun worshipper? If so, this might be the ideal time to give some advice about safer sun bathing.

2. Chemicals:
   - Has the patient developed a sudden rash around the area where a specific cream has been used?
   - Is the skin around a leg ulcer erythematous in the shape of a dressing?

Temperature regulation

The skin has a major role to play in regulating temperature. It is quite simple to observe and feel the skin, and skin temperature as measured by touch is a good initial indicator of body temperature, whether assessing for pyrexia or hypothermia.

Using the senses

When carrying out the assessment, it is worth remembering that four of the five senses can be used to gather information (Mairis, 1992):

1. Observation involves, quite obviously, looking for clues that indicate poor skin function. However, a complete visual assessment includes looking for non-verbal clues such as blushing due to embarrassment or shivering due to cold or fear.
2. Touch, which is discussed in more depth later, is crucial when giving psychological reassurance. It also gives a lot of physical clues, including detecting oedema by pressing the skin to see if it pits, checking temperature to see if the patient is especially hot or cold, and touching the skin to see how dry it is.
3. Smell is an assessment sense that nurses are probably unaware of using. However, it is usually obvious when patients are neglecting themselves and are not washing or changing their clothes, and certainly incontinence is often ascertained by smell rather than by patients admitting to it. Both these situations can have a detrimental effect on skin integrity. Certain infections of chronic wounds have characteristic smells; these will need investigating and possibly use of antibiotics following a positive skin swab.
4. Listening is the sense that it is hardest to see relevance for in terms of skin assessment. Paying careful attention to what is said by the patient is crucial, but it is also important to listen for involuntary sounds. These include cries of pain when a leg ulcer dressing is being changed, or the coos of delight when soothing moisturizers are applied to dry, cracked skin.

Describing skin lesions

When assessing the skin, it is useful to be able to describe the lesions that might be seen (Figure 1.1). Accurate descriptions can be useful aids to correct diagnosis. As nurses are more likely to see all areas of the skin, good descriptions provided to medical staff can mean speedier diagnosis of a lesion that may be dangerous – e.g. skin cancer. Using the terms also ensures that any changes are noticed and appropriate labels given. Skin lesions

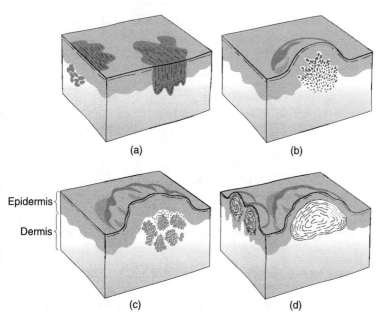

Epidermis

Dermis

Figure 1.1 Primary skin lesions: (a) macule (left, freckle; right, capillary haemangioma); (b) papule; (c) nodule; (d) bulla (left), vesicle (right).

can be broadly divided into two groups (de Witt, 1990); primary and secondary.

A primary lesion is the initial lesion developed by a patient with a skin problem, whereas a secondary lesion is one caused by the patient as a result of the primary condition. A secondary lesion might also be a primary lesion that has progressed and changed as a natural process (Delancy and North, 1983). For example, a primary lesion may well be a very itchy vesicle. The natural response is to scratch it, which may lead to secondary lesions called excoriations where the skin is broken through persistent scratching and trauma results.

Primary lesions

When describing a skin problem, it is helpful to use words that are more descriptive than 'a rash'. Table 1.2 provides a list of dermatological terms and their key characteristics. Even if you cannot find the right words to use, describing the location of the lesion, its size, colour, and whether it is wet or dry is a good start.

Table 1.2 Primary skin lesions: dermatological terms and key characteristics

Dermatological term	Description	Example
Macule (Fig. 1.1a)	Flat, various shapes, sizes and colours, usually hypo- or hyperpigmented	Vitiligo, freckles
Papule (Fig. 1.1b)	Small, solid, elevated, less than 1 cm in size	Warts, moles
Nodule (Fig. 1.1c)	Solid, elevated, 1–2 cm in size, extending into deeper tissues	Rheumatoid nodule
Weal/hive	Gently sloping, rounded or flat elevation several centimetres in size, may appear erythematous or pink	Usually in response to an allergic reaction
Vesicle (Fig. 1.1d)	Well-defined, fluid-filled, less than 0.5 cm in diameter	Chicken pox, poison ivy
Bulla (Fig. 1.1d)	Fluid-filled blister greater than 1 cm in diameter	Friction/thermal burns
Pustule	Elevated lesion, less than 1 cm diameter, containing pus visible through a translucent top	Acne
Cyst	Greater than 1 cm in diameter, containing semi-solid or liquid expressible material	Sebaceous cyst

Secondary lesions

Again it is useful to have some words to hand that describe the ways that primary lesions alter with time. Table 1.3 provides some examples.

Signs of secondary skin lesions also give some indication regarding the psychological status of a patient. The physical signs that indicate that someone has been scratching, give a good clue that the patient is uncomfortable and probably itchy. Thus the physical symptoms are useful as cues for assessment purposes.

Problem identification and goal setting

Problem identification and goal setting follow on from the assessment phase in the nursing process. Assessment data may be

Table 1.3 Secondary skin lesions: dermatological terms and key characteristics

Dermatological term	Description	Example
Excoriation	An abrasion in which loss of the epidermis occurs	Through scratching
Fissure	Crack through the epidermis and dermis as a result of very dry skin	
Lichenification	Thickening of the epidermis with increased skin markings	In eczema following extensive and prolonged scratching
Keloid	Elevated scar caused by excess collagen formation during the healing process	
Erythema	Blood vessels become dilated, causing redness and warmth	

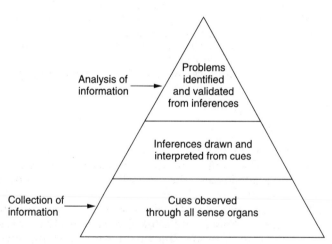

Figure 1.2 Identifying problems.

either subjective or objective in origin; subjective data include how a patient feels, whereas objective data are measurable and include measurement of vital signs. Figure 1.2 (Crow, 1979) illustrates how this data collection can then be used to identify problems.

The techniques and strategies identified earlier will help in achieving successful problem identification, which will in turn inform the planning of care. A problem correctly identified suggests that the present (or, on occasions, potential) situation is unsatisfactory for the patient. Identifying patient problems should, wherever possible, be a collaborative effort between the patient and the nurse. If patients are unable to express their needs, it is up to the nurse to use other sources such as family and friends along with his or her own skills to identify actual or potential problems.

Once problem areas have been identified, goal setting is necessary. Goals allow the monitoring of progress towards desired outcomes. For a goal statement to be effective, it should answer three key questions:

1. What change is to take place?
2. How will the change be observed?
3. When will the expected change be observed by?

The most effective goals are those that are realistically achievable and patient-focused. They are more likely to be realistic if they are divided into long- and short-term goals. For example, a long-term goal might be 'To have clear skin with no visible active psoriasis by the time of discharge'. Relevant short-term goals could then be 'To be able to apply moisturizers independently within 2 days of admission'; 'The skin will no longer be visibly scaling 1 week after admission'; and 'The centre of the plaques will be fading 8 days after admission'.

Planning care

A plan of care should logically flow from the goals, as it should be designed to achieve them. It should be carefully written in such a way that others can follow the plan in a logical fashion. The nursing actions required need to be clear so that anyone new to the patient's care will find guidance on what needs to be done. It is therefore useful if the points in the plan are numbered and clearly laid out. Any changes to the plan need to be clearly indicated and dated, and the original plan crossed through although remaining legible.

Patient focus is increased if patients are encouraged actively to participate in their care. This is especially relevant for those with a chronic longstanding skin problem, as they are likely to have previous knowledge and strategies for managing their disease. These need to be incorporated into goal-setting activities as well as planning care.

Implementation

It would be too simplistic to argue that once a plan of care is written implementation should follow in a straightforward way. The environment within which nurses practise, the resources they have available, the relationships they have with others and the training and education they have been able to undertake will all have a significant impact. Whilst close examination of each of these points is beyond the scope of this book, it is important to acknowledge them. Use of the nursing process and the other strategies highlighted in this chapter will assist in ensuring that a systematic approach is used so that no elements of care provision are omitted.

Evaluation

This phase of the nursing process has much in common with the assessment phase in that data are being collected regarding the patient – both objective and subjective. The main difference is that evaluation follows rather than precedes a nursing action, and involves making a judgement about patient progress towards a goal via a nursing action. Evaluation of patient care occurs on a day-to-day basis and is often documented at the end of a shift. However, effective evaluation requires more than a 'diary entry' of events for the patient during the shift. Evaluation should be used as:

- A measure of progress towards stated goals; these should be restated/reformulated if they have not been achieved by the agreed goal date
- An opportunity to identify new problems, which can be documented as part of the care plan.

Evaluation can therefore be seen as a form of reassessment, and reconfirms the view expressed earlier in this chapter that assessment has to be an ongoing process. To facilitate the process of evaluation, the SOAP mnemonic may be helpful:

S – subjective data
O – objective data
A – analysis
P – plan.

SOAP needs to be used in conjunction with a nursing care plan, and provides prompts to ensure that timely evaluation of patient problems occur. Thus rather than writing a diary-style entry at the end of the shift the nurse uses the SOAP mnemonic for each identified patient problem, considering the subjective and objective data collected during that shift and analysing whether the plan should be changed or carry on as already stated. If the plan is to stay the same, then the 'P' can in effect be ignored. The data collected in this way will facilitate the setting of goals that are relevant and meet the needs of patients.

The following example shows how this may work in reality. It only tackles one specific problem and should not be seen as a complete care plan, but it does give an idea as to how the SOAP mnemonic can be used.

Example

Celia Dowell has been admitted with a longstanding venous leg ulcer. She has said that the worse thing about it at the moment is the exudate, which means she has to put extra padding on once or twice a day after the district nurse has dressed it.

Problem: Heavily exuding wound, which soaks through three non-adherant pads per 24 hours.

Long-term goal: Reduce the exudate so that there is no strike through for 24 hours after the dressing has been done.

Short-term goals:

• Find a dressing that is comfortable (by the third day of admission)
• Mrs Dowell is to understand the importance of elevation to decrease exudate (by the third day of admission)
• There will be no need to put on extra padding (by the third day of admission).

Implementation:

• Dry leg well after soaking, especially between toes
• Apply Sorbsan Plus™ daily and secure with gauze and tubinette (see Chapter 3)
• Use Velband™ for padding
• Apply a compression bandage
• Encourage elevation with the foot of the bed raised.

Evaluation:

1. Day 1:

    S – Strikethrough occurred at 1800
    O – Says it is much more comfortable today

A – Still exuding excessively

P – Add extra padding for the night and change tomorrow morning.

2. Day 2:

S – Strikethrough occurred at 1500

O – Mrs Dowell says she does not like lying down with her legs elevated

A – Elevation is a problem

P – Advised Mrs Dowell of the importance of elevation and put extra pillows on bed to make her more comfortable. Extra padding applied to the leg, to be changed tomorrow morning.

3. Day 3:

S – No strikethrough at 21.30

O – Mrs Dowell is delighted and says she feels much more comfortable

A – Elevation achieved and Sorbsan Plus™ suits

P – Goal achieved, no extra plan.

Three core themes

Having outlined strategies for planning care for someone with a skin problem, it is useful to give consideration to some core themes. These themes are relevant to all areas of nursing, but because of the nature of skin as a tactile organ and one of display, they are even more pertinent. Thus the themes addressed here will be familiar to you, but there is benefit in further thought in the context of caring for someone with altered skin function.

Privacy

Looking after the skin means that the nurse will have close physical contact with patients' bodies. It is more than likely that patients will need to remove their clothes to allow for assessment or treatment of their skin. Being naked in front of a stranger is likely to cause discomfort to most people, and this can be exacerbated to acute embarrassment if they have a skin disease that they perceive to be unsightly or disfiguring. Whilst strategic covering of certain 'private' areas may be possible (as in a bed bath), this is often not possible in reality because these areas are affected by the skin disease.

Lawler (1991) carried out an extensive research study on how nurses respond to patients' bodies. Her work helps us to understand the body and how nurses and patients cope with the intrusions that are not normal in everyday existence. She identifies that the body is not just an object but allows us to have a presence amongst others and gives us a personal identity. The body is part of our lived experience and patients with skin problems will be acutely aware of how they appear and their personal identity may be seriously undermined.

The nurse can, by his or her behaviour, make the experience of exposure less embarrassing. Ensuring that disturbances will not occur is a simple way. If a patient is going to be asked to strip off completely, doing this in a bathroom where the door can be locked rather than behind flimsy curtains may be reassuring. Lawler (1991) spends some time examining the concept of privacy as understood by nurses. It is clear from her work that privacy is not just about a lack of audience; it is also about 'ensuring no unnecessary body exposure, minimizing the possibility of embarrassment, maintaining dignity for a person and an aspect of personhood'. Therefore whilst a locked door is a sensible, practical way of ensuring privacy, it is more complex than this. Some skin conditions can be unsightly to look at, and a nurse can help patients to feel less embarrassed by ensuring that his or her reaction is not a negative one. Saying how awful someone's skin looks is not reassuring, even if the patient is well aware of the fact. This last point is very important. When talking to people with skin disease, it becomes very clear how conscious they are of how others react to their visible disease. The reaction does not even have to be particularly overt for it to be potentially hurtful.

Touch

It is unlikely that embarrassment will be the only emotion that patients feel when they come into hospital. Anxiety on admission to hospital is well documented, and historically the solution to this has been to ensure that good information is given (Hayward, 1975; Boore, 1978; Wilson Barnett, 1978). However, as Teasdale (1995) suggests, there are many other strategies that can be implemented to reduce anxiety. One of the key strategies in relation to people with skin problems is support using closeness and touch. Touch is one of the most universal ways of showing caring (Sundeen *et al.*, 1989), and when someone has a skin problem touch is increasingly important to allay the fear of being untouchable and in some way contagious (skin diseases are very rarely contagious). Touch can be used in a number of ways to help patients (see below); however, Sayre-Adams and Wright (1995) point out that for touch to be effective it must be 'authentically given by a warm, genuine caring individual to one who is willing to receive it'. This becomes even more important because those with skin problems are so acutely sensitive; unthinking, careless touch can be physically painful and emotionally unhelpful.

Four broad categories of touch can be identified, all of which have their place when caring for someone with skin problems:

1. Instrumental touch involves deliberative physical contact used to perform some physical task, e.g. application of a topical steroid.
2. Expressive touch is a more spontaneous gesture that is not related to a specific task and might be used for comfort or reassurance, e.g. holding someone's hand whilst he tells you about the death of a loved one.
3. Therapeutic touch is more complex to describe. It is a specific type of touch, and is thus denoted by using initial upper-case letters when writing about it. It has been defined by Malinski (1993) as 'a health patterning modality whereby nurse and client participate knowingly in the changing human–environmental field process'. It has also been described as a non-religious laying-on of hands, which involves the realignment of energy flow round a client/patient by moving the hands above the body.
4. There are other forms of touch that are said to be therapeutic but are not the Therapeutic touch. These include practices such as massage, reflexology and acupuncture.

Autonomy

Many skin conditions are chronic in nature and therefore patients have coped with them for years. Nurses need to bear this in mind when planning care to ensure that the patient's autonomy is maintained. It may well be that individuals have already established a skin care routine that works for them. If this is the case, during the assessment this must be noted and care plans written accordingly. For example, if a patient usually has a bath every day, this needs to be accommodated. Conversely, people with chronic skin conditions are sometimes just so glad to have someone else to help them with their skin care that they would gladly relinquish any responsibility for caring for their own skin (Kirkevold, 1993). If this is the case, plans of care should be made to meet these immediate needs, but also include plans for the future when the individuals take back responsibility for looking after themselves.

Allowing patients to discuss the issues that are worrying them, finding out what their fears are and then empowering them to get over these fears is a way of increasing their feeling of autonomy and therefore reducing anxiety. If patients have confidence in the nursing staff who look after them, this is in turn likely to boost their own confidence levels as well as their self worth and personal coping abilities (Kirk, 1992). Thus patients need to have confidence in their carer so that they trust the care they are receiving. This care can be enhanced by using touch and ensuring that patients have relevant and understandable information. The above is summarized well by Sundeen *et al.* (1989) when they describe the nurse–patient relationship as:

> *. . . learning experiences whereby two people interact to face an immediate health problem, to share if possible, in resolving it and to discover ways to adapt to the situation.*

Conclusion

In summary, three key themes need to be kept in mind when planning care for someone with altered skin function:

1. Privacy – how this is going to be maintained, how much of the person's body is going to be exposed, and how this will make the patient feel
2. Touch – how the most relevant type of touch can be used to help patients
3. Autonomy – this is promoted through empowerment (particularly through good information giving) and encouraging self care.

Whilst these issues are relevant to all fields of nursing and all types of patient, they take on a special importance for a patient with skin problems because of the necessity of exposure. Coming to terms with the feelings that this engenders (both for the nurse and the patient) is essential if holistic care is to be given.

Reflective activities

1. Consider the judgements that you make every day, both in your professional and in your social life, just by looking at someone's skin.
2. Think back to early in your nursing career and remember the first occasion you came across nudity of a patient. How did it

make you feel? How did you react to the situation? What sort of support were you offered, or were you just expected to 'get on with it'? Reflect on how we learn to cope with this sort of exposure, which would never occur in our social lives.

3. Consider the most commonly occurring medical conditions on your ward or unit. Read around the topic, if necessary, and make lists of any part that the skin has to play in these conditions.

4. Once you have done the above, think about the patient problems associated with the skin involvement. Keep this work, and complete model patient care plans once you have read the remaining chapters in this book.

5. Think about a strategy for incorporating skin assessment into your everyday practice. Once you have got some initial ideas, discuss these with colleagues and formalize a plan of action.

References

Bore, R. P. (1978). *Prescription for Recovery*. RCN.

Crow, J. (1979). Assessment. In: *The Nursing Process* (C. R. Kratz, ed.), pp. Bailliere Tindall.

de Witt, S. (1990). Nursing assessment of skin and dermatologic lesions. *Nursing Clin. North Am.*, **25(1)**, 235–45.

Delancy, V. L. and North, C. (1983). Skin assessment topics. *Clinical Nursing*, **5(2)**, 5–10.

Doenges, M. E. and Moorhouse, M. F. (1992). *Application of Nursing Process and Nursing Diagnosis: An Interactive Text*. F. A. Davis.

Hayward, J. (1975). *Information: Prescription against Pain*. RCN.

Kirk, K. (1992). Confidence as a factor in chronic illness care. *J. Adv. Nursing*, **17(10)**, 1238–42.

Kirkevold, M. (1993). Toward a practice theory of caring for patient with chronic skin disease. *Scholarly inquiry for Nursing Practice*, **7(1)**, 37–52.

Lawler, J. (1991). *Behind the Screens – Nursing, Somology and the Problem of the Body*. Churchill Livingstone.

Mairis, E. (1992). Four senses for a full skin assessment. *Prof. Nurse*, **7(6)**, 376–8.

Malinski, V. (1993). Therapeutic Touch: the view from Rogerian Nursing Science Visions. *J. Rogerian Nursing Sci.*, **1(1)**, 45–54.

Orem, D. E. (1985). A concept of self-care for the rehabilitation client. *Rehab. Nursing*, **10(3)**, 33–6.

Roy, C. (1988). An explication of the philosophical assumptions of the Roy adaptation model. *Nursing Sci. Q.*, **1(1)**, 26–34.

Sayre-Adams, J. and Wright, S. (1995). *The Theory and Practice of Therapeutic Touch*. Churchill Livingstone.

Sundeen, S. J., Stuart, G. W., Rankin, E. A. D. and Cohen, S. A. (1989). *Nurse–Client Interaction – Implementing the Nursing Process*, 4th edn. CV Mosby Co.

Teasdale, R. (1995). Theoretical and practical considerations on the use of reassurance in the nursing management of anxious patients. *J. Adv. Nurs.*, **22(1)**, 79–86.

UKCC Guidelines on Record Keeping, Factors influencing patients emotion of reactions to hospitalisation. *J. Adv. Nurs.*, **3(3)**, 221–9.

Wilson Barnett. (1978). www.ukcc.org.uk

Normal skin: its function and care

Fiona Pringle and Rebecca Penzer

Introduction

The focus of this chapter is on normal skin. Skin alters as we go through life, and what is normal for a child will not necessarily be so for an older person. Normal skin from a sociological viewpoint can be considered through issues of body image (these are discussed further in Chapter 4). Normal skin function from a biological perspective can be explained by looking at structure and function and examining whether these fall within normal parameters.

This chapter considers the structure and function of the skin; skin at different stages of life, including problems affecting particular age groups; caring for the skin of those without a specific skin condition; and the differences between black and white skin.

Structure and function of the skin

It is important that nurses understand what the normal parameters of skin function and structure are before going on to consider the skin when it is functioning outside these parameters. This understanding needs to be within the context of patient care, and thus this chapter covers the biology of the structure and function of the skin but also looks at some key factors to consider when caring for patients. This chapter presumes that the patient does not have skin disease, and examines how good skin care can be promoted.

Although human beings are relatively naked compared to other mammals they do still have head hair, which has remained to provide protection from the sun and minor injuries. They have also developed a unique combination of features within the skin: thick outer layers, a widespread system of thermal sensitive sweat glands, and an extensive layer of fatty tissue at the undersurface of the skin. This complex arrangement allows humans to survive in a wide range of environmental conditions (Morris, 1977).

The skin is the body's largest organ, making up about 15 per cent of the total body weight. It is not uniformly the same in all areas of the body, the differences depending upon the function of the specific area. For example, skin thickness varies; on the eyelid it is only 0.5 mm thick, whilst on the soles of the feet it may be as much as 3–4 mm thick (Brooker, 1998). This thickening of the skin may in part be due to the intermittent pressure that is exerted on the soles of the feet and the palms of the hands.

Structure of the skin

Broadly speaking, the skin consists of the epidermis and the dermis. The epidermis is the outermost layer and is responsible for most of the skin's protective functions. Below the epidermis lies the dermis, the function of which is to support the epidermis (Figure 2.1).

The epidermis

The epidermis is a multi-layered structure that regularly renews itself through cell division in its deepest layer (Figure 2.2). It can vary in thickness from 0.1 mm over the eyelid to over 1 mm on the soles of the feet. It does not contain any blood vessels.

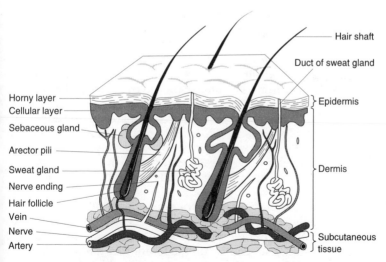

Figure 2.1 A cross-section of the dermis and epidermis
(Courtesy of Walsh *et al.*, 2001).

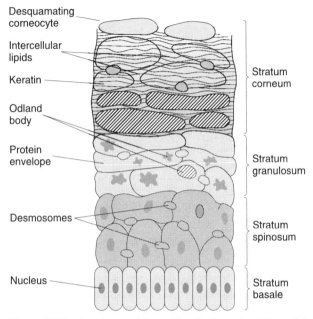

Figure 2.2 The four layers of the epidermis (figure is not to scale).

Stratum basale (basal cell layer)

The basal cell layer, or undersurface, is composed of two distinct types of cells; keratinocytes and melanocytes. The keratinocytes' function relates to the development of the stratum corneum, i.e. the top layer of the epidermis. Melanocytes, as their name suggests, are responsible for the production of melanin, which protects the skin from the damage caused by ultraviolet radiation. The basal cells form the germinative pool and, under normal circumstances, are the only epidermal cells capable of division. Each basal cell divides to form two daughter cells, thus doubling the number of cells. Each cell divides approximately every 19 days. Following cell division, the daughter cells then begin moving towards the skin's surface. This usually takes about 28 days.

Stratum spinosum (prickle cell or squamous cell layer)

As the daughter cell moves into this layer it loses its ability to divide and it becomes more rounded in shape. This layer is 5–12 cells in thickness, depending on the location in the body. It is the squamous cell layer that gives rise to the mechanical bulk of the epidermis. Each daughter cell is an individual cell and is joined to other daughter cells by intracellular bridges called desmosomes. It is these intracellular bridges that give the prickle cell layer its name, as they have been compared to the prickles on a seed. As the daughter cell moves through the squamous cell layer it is constantly breaking and reforming the desmosomes.

Stratum granulosum

As the cells migrate towards the surface of the skin they elongate and flatten horizontally to form the stratum granulosum. Great metabolic changes occur and it is in this process that the squamous cells lose all their intracellular machinery, including the nuclei. The cell is now composed almost entirely of a tough, pliable protein called keratin. At this stage Odland bodies are seen; these granules contain lipid, which extrudes into the intercellular spaces and help the cells to 'stick' together.

Stratum corneum (horny layer)

This is the final layer in the structure of the epidermis. The cells of the horny layer are arranged in orderly vertical stacks, and appear to be composed of cell membranes each firmly attached to one another. The cells are dead by this stage. The cell membranes consist of soft keratin, which helps to keep the skin elastic and protects the living cells underneath from exposure to the air and drying out. The intercellular lipid from the stratum granulosum cements the cells together and is crucial in preventing epidermal desiccation. As the cells move through the stratum corneum they lose their cohesion and are shed singly or in clumps.

Each of the four levels in the epidermis represents a stage in the life of an epidermal cell. Since the horny layer forms the final barrier between the body and the often harsh environment, it is subject to considerable wear and tear and for this reason must have a means of regular renewal. As already shown, the epidermis achieves this renewal by producing a pool of proliferative cells that migrate from the basal layer to the environment in approximately 28 days, of which at least 14 days are spent in the horny layer.

Although the dead cells of the horny layer are constantly shedding, under normal circumstances this process does not provide enough scales to become noticeable. In order for the skin to maintain appropriate thickness and important barrier functions, there must be a constant balance between the formation of new keratinocytes by division of the basal cells and the rate of falling off of the dead keratinocytes from the outermost stratum corneum. If dead skin cells fall off faster than new cells are formed, then the skin becomes thin, eroded or atrophic. If new cells are formed faster than dead cells are sloughed off, then the stratum corneum piles up and appears as scales or thickened skin.

The epidermis and the dermis are joined together by the dermal papillae. These structures ensure the layers of skin are held together; trauma or shearing forces can cause them to separate, leading to blister formation.

The dermis

Whereas the epidermis functions as the barrier between the body and the environment, the dermis functions to support the epidermis structurally and nutritionally and lies between the epidermis and the subcutaneous fat layer. The dermis also contains lymph vessels, nerve endings, hair follicles and glands.

Composition of the dermis

The dermis consists of two distinct layers, the reticular and papillary layers. The papillary layer contains the nerves and capillaries that supply the epidermal layer, whilst the more dense reticular layer provides strength through collagen and elastin. The interwoven fibres of collagen and elastin, packed in bundles, make up the bulk of the dermis.

Collagen is a protein that makes up about 70 per cent of the dry weight of the dermis. It is a long molecule woven together in such a way as to allow stretching and contraction while still maintaining its tensile strength. Collagen is the major source of the mechanical strength of the skin. When the skin is stretched, the collagen, with its high tensile strength, prevents tearing.

Elastin fibres are also synthesized by fibroblasts. These are finer than collagen and are found intertwined among the collagen bundles. As its name suggests, elastin has elastic properties and its function is to return the skin to its normal position following stretching.

Elastin and collagen bundles at any particular points of the body tend to be organized in parallel bundles known as lines of tension (Martini, 1998). A cut in the skin made parallel to these lines of tension will not gape, as the collagen and elastin will ensure that the opposing edges hold together. However, an incision made across the lines of tension will cut through the collagen and elastin bundles so that they cannot hold together opposing edges, and the wound will therefore gape, bleed and scar to a much greater extent.

The amorphous ground substance of the dermis consists mainly of glycosaminoglycans, a complex amino acid. The ground substance has three important functions:

1. It binds water, allowing nutrients, hormones and waste products to pass through the dermis. However, its thick 'syrupy' consistency makes it hard for bacteria to move through it.
2. It is a lubricant between the collagen and elastic fibre networks during skin movement.
3. It provides bulk, allowing the dermis to act as a shock absorber.

Glands in the dermis

1. *Sweat glands.* There are two types of sweat glands. The eccrine glands produce sweat, which consists mainly of water, to ensure that the body is able to thermoregulate. Apocrine glands are non-active in childhood, but appear to be activated by sex hormones because they become active at puberty. This supports the view that their function has an influence on sexual behaviour. They are found mainly in the axillae, around the nipples and in the ano-genital area, and secrete a sticky odourless substance. This substance is rapidly acted on by bacteria, thus creating a smell most commonly known as body odour. Their structure is better developed in the Afro-Caribbean population and less well developed amongst Asians.
2. *Sebaceous glands.* The oily secretion from these glands is made up of cholesterol and other lipids, and is called sebum. Sebaceous glands (which can either secrete into a hair follicle or directly onto the skin) are most numerous on the face, neck and back. Sebum acts as lubricant and protector for the skin, creating a permeable barrier that has antibacterial and fungicidal properties. Sebaceous glands are especially active in the teenage years, stimulated by the action of androgens. Acne, caused by bacterial action on sebum leading to blocked follicles, inflammation and infection, is usual to some degree in teenagers. Sebum production is less in the very young and old, thus skin care at these two age extremes is especially important, as the body's ability to protect the skin is diminished.

Blood vessels

There are two main networks of cutaneous arteries. The deep plexus is at the junction of the dermis and the subcutaneous fat layer and supplies subcutaneous and dermal tissues. Smaller arteries branch away from this towards the epidermis and supply the hair follicles, sweat glands and other structures of the dermis. On reaching the papillary dermis a second branching network occurs, called the superficial or papillary plexus. This supplies capillary blood vessels at the epidermis–dermis boundary. The capillaries empty into small veins, which connect to larger veins in the subcutaneous layer.

Skin appendages

Hair and nails are part of the skin, and are made up of different types of keratin.

Hair

Hair has some protective qualities, for example on the head for protection from the sun and trauma, and the eyebrows and eyelashes to protect the eyes, but in comparison with other mammals humans are relatively naked. Hair – either too much or not enough – has a major impact on the perception of sexual attractiveness, and as such is of importance in the portrayal of a self-image.

The apparatus for hair growth can be found in the dermis or extending into the subcutaneous layer. It consists of a follicle, which has a region from which the hair grows known as the bulb, and the hair itself, which has a root and a shaft. The arrector pili muscle is connected to the follicle and is responsible for the goose bumps experienced in the cold or times of extreme fright. When the muscle contracts the hairs stand on end and are more able to trap a layer of warm air next to the body, thus conserving heat. This is not a particularly effective mechanism for heat conservation due to the sparse and fine nature of human body hair.

Adults have two types of hair. Vellus hair describes the small hairs located all over the body, and these make up 98 per cent of the five million hairs that cover the body. Terminal hairs are more deeply pigmented – eyelashes, eyebrows and head hair all fall into this category. All hair follicles have active and resting periods; during the resting period the old hair drops out before the new one starts growing. Throughout life, hair follicles become more or less active depending on where they are located. The follicles on the head become less active for both sexes, causing thinning of the hair. On average an adult loses 50 hairs from the head every day, and sustained loss of 100 or more hairs per day usually indicates that something is wrong – e.g. excess of vitamin A, high fever or stress.

Nails

Nails are made of sheets of keratin and are comparable to the hoofs and claws of animals. Their tough nature makes them ideal for protecting the ends of the fingers and enables humans to perform very delicate movements. They grow from a number of germinative cells known as the nail root, which is not visible to the eye. The very tip of the finger under the growth of the nail is the hyponychium (Figure 2.3), which is an area of thickened stratum corneum for greater protection of the digit ends. Nail beds are usually pink in colour because of the extensive capillary network beneath the nail, and discoloured nails can be indicative of disease (Spindler and Data, 1992).

Functions of the skin

The skin uses its complex structure to perform a number of different functions.

Sensory perception

Touch is one of the most important senses. The body is able to react to external stimuli such as cold, heat, pain, touch and pressure. This makes the skin an important organ of sensory perception. The skin is supplied with approximately one million nerve fibres, most of which end in the face and extremities. These nerves have different functions, and can be classified according to these functions or according to their structure (Table 2.1).

On responding to stimuli, these receptors relay the data to the central nervous system. When necessary the central nervous system reacts, causing a mechanical response – e.g. pulling your hand away from an electric fence touched by mistake.

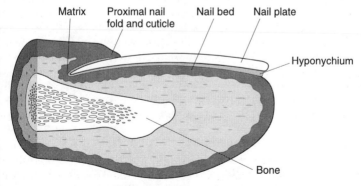

Figure 2.3 Structure of a nail.

Table 2.1 Sensory perception in the skin

Stimulus	Structure	Function
Pain	Free dendritic nerve endings	Nocioreceptors
Touch	Free dendritic nerve endings	Mechanoreceptors
Temperature	Free dendritic nerve endings	Thermoreceptors
Pressure	Encapsulated receptors (light pressure)	Mechanoreceptors
	Free dendritic nerve endings (other pressure)	

Thermoregulation

The skin plays an important part in the body's system for maintaining a relatively constant internal temperature in the face of highly variable outside temperatures. Receptors in the skin monitor temperature and transmit impulses to central control mechanisms in the hypothalamus. This responds by manipulating the cutaneous vessels, muscles and eccrine sweat glands, along with other metabolic functions such as respiratory and heart rates, to keep the body's core temperature constant.

Cutaneous mechanisms of temperature control include insulation, sweating and regulation of blood flow.

Insulation
Insulation is provided by subcutaneous adipose tissue found under the dermis. Further detail about the function of this layer is provided in the section on the storage function of the skin (see below).

Sweating
Sweating as a method of thermoregulation is rather more involved. There are two types of sweat glands. The apocrine glands have little to do with thermoregulation (see the section on the dermis for further detail). The eccrine glands are those that produce sweat, and they do this when the temperature rises above 37°C. They are most profuse on the palms of the hands and soles of the feet. In these areas there are up to 500 cm² (Martini, 1998) compared to on the back, where there are a mere 70 cm². There is always some water loss through the lungs, for example, known as insensible loss, which reaches 400–500 ml/day. Normal perspiration causes the loss of about a further 400 ml/day. However, in hot climates and during vigorous exercise water loss through sweating may rise to 12 000 ml/day. Sweat cools the

body because heat energy is required to evaporate it from the body. This latent heat energy is gained from the surface of the skin. Thermal sweating is a reflex response to a raised environmental temperature and occurs all over the body, but especially in the chest, back, forehead, scalp and axillae.

The above discussion indicates how sweating occurs because of thermal changes. It is however, common to experience sweating as a result of two further stimuli; emotion and spicy food. Emotional sweating is provoked mostly by fear and anxiety, and occurs mainly on the palms, soles and axillae. Gustatory sweating is provoked by hot, spicy foods, and affects the face.

Regulation of cutaneous blood flow

The skin has an abundant blood supply, which allows regulation of body temperature. The core temperature within the body needs to remain constant. Thus if the external temperature rises, the body responds by increasing the blood flow to the skin so that more body heat is moved towards the surface of the skin where it can be dissipated. Conversely, when the body's core temperature needs to be conserved, the blood vessels constrict, so keeping the warm blood within the main internal organs and minimalizing the amount lost to the atmosphere through peripheral blood flow. Therefore, the skin appears red when the body is overheated as the blood vessels are dilated to allow an increase in blood flow at the skin's surface, and white when the body is cold as the blood vessels contract to conserve heat (Rook *et al.*, 1979) (Figure 2.4).

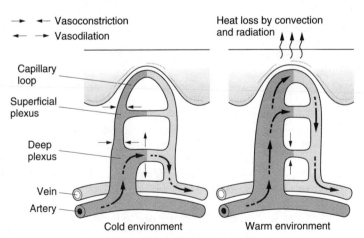

Figure 2.4 Variations in the skin's blood supply under cold and warm conditions.

It is the ability of the blood vessels in the skin to contract and dilate and so increase or decrease the amount of blood at the skin's surface that determines the amount of heat lost. Heat may be lost from the skin in three ways: through radiation, which means the heat moves directly into the surrounding air; through conduction, which allows heat to be lost through an object (e.g. a chair or bed); and finally through convection, where warm currents of air are moved away from the body to be replaced by cooler ones.

Protection

Since human beings are exposed to heat, cold, water, trauma, friction and pressure, the skin must be durable. It must also be pliable, because humans are active and mobile and use many delicate motions. The skin must be strong enough to be protective, yet sensitive enough to relay important messages about our environment.

The skin acts as a physical protective barrier for the internal organs, shielding them from damage and preventing harmful micro-organisms and foreign substances entering the body (Cork, 1997). Whilst acting as an insulator keeping the environment within the body at a relatively constant temperature, the skin also prevents fluid loss. Besides sweat, there is very little transfer of water across the skin, which prevents the internal organs from drying out. Because it is dry bacterial proliferation is discouraged, and the skin's constantly shedding nature means that micro-organisms do not get chance to 'take hold'. The secretions onto the surface of the skin tend to be acidic in nature, acting as an antibacterial agent and offering further protection (Brooker, 1998).

The skin's complex structure means that it can protect the body not only by virtue of its physical presence as described above, but also through biological processes that occur in it. Examples of this include protection from the sun as light is absorbed by melanin pigment, and the triggering of an immunological response when the physical barrier of the skin is breached by bacteria. This immunological response is initiated by the presence of antigens on the surface of bacteria or other foreign bodies. Specialized dendritic cells, called Langerhans cells, which are thought to be related to the monocyte/macrophage system, are important at this point. Langerhans cells only exist in skin, maturing into such from dendritic cells once they leave the circulatory system and enter the skin tissues. Unlike macrophages, Langerhans cells are not phagocytic. Instead they function by attracting antigens and then presenting them to T lymphocytes, thus activating the lymphocytes to kill relevant cells. It is recognized that Langerhans cells (and dendritic cells in general) have a crucial role to play between the antigens (and antigen recognition) and the adaptive immune system (i.e. lymphocytes) (Davies, 1997).

Synthesis of vitamin D

Vitamin D is essential for skeletal development, and it is synthesized in the skin as a result of exposure to ultraviolet B light. The vitamin controls the amount of calcium and phosphorus absorbed through the small intestine and mobilized from bone. The amount of melanin in the skin affects the exposure time required to synthesize the vitamin. In order to maximize the levels of previtamin D, black skin needs 12 times the length of exposure to UVB as white skin. This is probably due to the fact that only 2–5 per cent of incident UVB penetrates through the epidermis in Afro-Caribbean people compared to 20–30 per cent in Caucasians. This method of vitamin D production is only of limited importance in Britain, as most vitamin D is provided in the diet (Holick *et al.*, 1981).

Storage

In physiologically challenging situations such as starvation or dehydration the skin acts as a store for water; specifically, the subcutaneous adipose tissues act as a fat reserve which can be utilized to produce energy. There are three key factors that determine the amount and type of fat stored:

1. The genes that are inherited from parents, which determine an individual's bulk.
2. Whether an individual is male or female; females tend to have a greater percentage of adipose tissue.
3. The age of an individual – older people have less adipose tissue, which means they have less effective insulation and reduced ability to survive in periods of starvation or dehydration. Babies have a type of fat (brown fat) that yields energy more readily than other fat cells; they are well insulated, as the proportion of fat in their body weight is greater than for adults.

Psychological

The skin plays an essential role in the psychological well-being of a person. It is the organ of display, and when it goes wrong the consequences can be anxiety, withdrawal and embarrassment. Shuster (1981) reminds us how socially unacceptable skin disease is. It seems possible that our profound and almost instinctive loathing of diseased skin (a response that is out of all proportion to the objective manifestation) stems from an association with contagious infestation and infection common in historical societies. The treatment of lepers in biblical times is an excellent example of how those with skin lesions became ostracized and outcast from communities. In contrast, if the skin looks good it can engender a feeling of well-being – for example, many people would say that they feel better with a suntan, although in reality the suntan does the biology of their skin very few favours.

When the skin performs its functions normally, we see it only in terms of its cosmetic, aesthetic value, its racial significance and its contribution towards non-verbal communication. However, if any of the cutaneous mechanisms malfunction, we suffer discomfort, disfigurement and possible death (Hunter *et al.*, 1995).

Skin through the ages

Skin quality varies throughout the age spectrum. What may be normal during childhood is not necessarily so later on in life.

Skin in childhood

There are some specific conditions that relate to normal skin during childhood development. At birth the skin is frequently covered with a white greasy substance, the vernix caseosa. In mature babies it is usually only found in the skin creases, but it may also cover the trunk of those babies who are pre-term. It is secreted by the fetal sebaceous glands, and protects the skin from its watery environment *in utero*. Post-mature babies have lost this protective covering and thus tend to have dry, peeling skin. Further protection from the watery intrauterine environment is provided by the growth of lanugo, a type of hair that falls out soon after birth to be replaced by vellus and terminal hair.

Milia

Many babies develop tiny white spots called milia over their nose and face, and these are caused by blocked sebaceous glands. The formation of milia may be related to hormone stimulus of the sebaceous glands. These glands gradually become smaller and inactive after birth, and remain quiescent until adolescence. As the sebaceous glands become less active, the milia disappear. Milia should never be squeezed or pinched (Neff and Spray, 1996).

Erythema toxicum

This non-infective rash is of unknown origin, develops within a day or two of birth, and resolves spontaneously. It presents as whitish/yellowish papules or pustules that are no more than 3 mm in size.

Icterus neonatorum (physiologic jaundice)

A couple of days after birth the newborn may become yellowish in colour. This is quite normal, and is a result of the breakdown of the excess red blood cells the infant needed when *in utero*. Once respiration occurs following birth there is no longer the need for the extra red blood cells, and the cell breakdown leads to high serum bilirubin levels and the consequent yellow colour. (*NB*: the appearance of jaundice within 24 hours of birth is known as pathologic jaundice, and may be indicative of rhesus or ABO incompatibilities.)

Mongolian blue spot

A Mongolian blue spot may be present on the lower back of a baby of East Asian or Afro-Caribbean parents. The spot is usually present at birth, and resembles a blue bruise over the sacral area. The blue-black colour is caused by elongated melanocyte precursor cells in the lower dermis. The spot usually disappears as the child grows older, but some remain into adulthood. The presence of a Mongolian blue spot must always be documented in the nursing and medical notes, as it can be mistaken for bruising caused by non-accidental injury.

Nevus flammeus (port-wine stain)

Port-wine stains are caused by a capillary angioma located just below the epidermis, and are generally not elevated. They often appear on the face and tend not to increase or decrease in size with time. In Afro-Carribean skin they are jet-black in colour; in white skin they are red.

Telangiectatic naevus (strawberry birthmark)

Strawberry naevi are vascular lesions formed by the dilation of a group of small blood vessels. They are red in colour, but usually resolve spontaneously as the child matures.

Freckles

Freckles are flat, well-circumscribed brown lesions scattered over sun-exposed areas, and thus are not present in newborn infants or young children. Freckles are caused by local groups of melanocytes that are genetically determined to be more sensitive to solar radiation than those of the surrounding skin, and therefore they do not occur without sun exposure. They are harmless.

Children and the sun

Children have more delicate skin than adults and are therefore more sun-sensitive. They also spend more time out in the sun wearing less clothing and at inappropriate times when the sun is at its most intense – for example, during school lunch breaks. Skin cancers in later life may occur because of the skin damage caused in childhood – the more sinister effects of sunburn do not manifest themselves until later life – and it is therefore important to protect children with densely woven cotton T-shirts and wide-brimmed hats, and to keep them out of the sun between 11 am and 3 pm. Babies under the age of 6 months should be kept out of the sun altogether. It is estimated that around 80 per cent of solar damage to the skin occurs during childhood, so it makes sense for parents to get into the habit of applying sunscreen as part of their normal routine (Perkins, 1993).

Ultraviolet light B (UVB) is a short-wave light band (290–350 nm) and penetrates the epidermis, whilst ultraviolet light A (UVA) is a long-wave light band (320–400 nm) and penetrates through to the dermis. UVB rays are responsible for causing burning and tanning of the skin, and UVA rays are responsible for the ageing effect of sunlight. Protection against UVB rays, which cause redness and burning, are a first priority, and children should be encouraged to use a sunscreen with a high sun protection factor (SPF). High protection numbers are SPF15 and above, but the SPF does not indicate the level of UVA protection. A star rating system has been devised that measures the degree of UVA protection. The ideal aim is to reduce the levels of UVA and UVB equally so that exposure to one is not greater than to the other (Morton,

1993), and therefore the higher the SPF chosen, the higher the equivalent star rating should be. There are four categories of star rating, and the more stars the higher the protection, so if possible choose a product that offers at least SPF15 and a three-star rating.

Puberty

At puberty, the gonads begin to secrete hormones that cause the genitals to grow and the secondary sexual characteristics to appear. The skin also responds. Androgens stimulate maturation and secretory activity of hair follicles and sebaceous glands in certain body areas. At this time of stimulation of hair growth, the incidence of occlusion, irritation and infection of hair follicles increases.

Acne

It is hard to decide whether acne should be incorporated into this chapter or the next. However, in view of the fact that nearly all teenagers suffer from some form of acne in their lives, it would seem to be a normal part of growing up. Having said this, it is acknowledged that there is nothing normal about the degree of acne that some people experience, and by putting it in this chapter it is in no way diminishing the adverse impact that it can have on people's lives.

The sebaceous glands of the face, chest and upper back become large and functional, and it is at this time that acne may develop. Acne is the most common disease of the skin, and develops when sebum excretion is increased due to stimulation by the androgens. The increased oiliness of the skin can cause the epithelium to overgrow the follicular surface and so occlude the follicle, causing retention of sebum. This in turn causes an increase in the concentration of bacteria and free fatty acids within the follicle. Products from the bacteria contribute to further follicular epithelial changes and lead to comedone (blackhead) and whitehead formation. Other products destroy leukocytes and initiate the inflammation characteristic of acne (Black, 1995).

Acne affects the sexes equally. It usually first affects adolescents between the ages of 12 and 14 years, tending to be earlier in females. The peak age and severity is 16–17 years in females and 17–19 in males. However, acne can occur in much younger children and in older adults too. At some time during puberty most teenagers will suffer some degree of acne, and it is only a minority that develop severe acne in which nodules form and lesions coalesce and occasionally form sinus tracts (Black, 1995).

Whatever the physical degree of acne, it is important to take into account how individuals are coping with their acne and how they feel about it. It is not a trivial problem that they should 'grow out of', but one that can have profound effects on their lives (Carroll, 2000). Acne can be extremely distressing, leading to isolation and low self-esteem in what is a vulnerable developmental stage of life.

Acne is treatable; however, for treatments to be successful they need to be tried over a period of time before changing or moving on to something new. This can be distressing for the person involved, who will need a lot of support and encouragement.

For mild acne, preparations bought over the counter are often sufficient. Benzoyl peroxide is usually the active ingredient, and comes in 2.5 per cent, 5 per cent and 10 per cent strengths. People should always start with the lower strengths, as the 10 per cent in particular can cause soreness and dryness. If after a 2–3-month trial these are not sufficient to control the acne, the next step is antibiotics, erythromycin and tetracyclines being those of choice. Advice should be given about taking the tetracyclines 1 hour before food for therapeutic efficacy. In girls, the introduction of cypoterone acetate (Dianette™) should be considered at this stage.

Referral to a dermatologist may be necessary, and the National Institute for Clinical Excellence guidelines makes several recommendations (including urgent referral for those with severe acne); however, they also recommend routine referrals for those who are showing signs of scarring and those who do not respond to two 3-month courses of antibiotics (NICE, 2000). A dermatologist will be able to offer further advice and may prescribe isotretin (Roaccutane™). Isotretin is a synthetic derivative of vitamin A, and has a profound suppressive effect on the sebaceous glands. This drug can only be prescribed from hospitals and has a number of potential side effects, including teratogenicity (Novotny, 1989).

It is important to reassure teenagers that acne is not caused by poor diet, eating chocolate or being dirty. Such reassurance may help youngsters to cope with the unpleasant peer pressure they experience. Nurses can also help by providing practical guidance, such as keeping the skin clean but not over-washing. The skin should be cleansed no more than twice a day with a non-soap facial wash and then patted dry. If a topical treatment is being used it should be applied at this stage, and it should be put on all over the affected area not just dabbed onto the spots. Make-up can be worn, but it should be non-oily (non-comodogenic) and applied about 20 minutes after the topical treatment (if this is being used).

Many people with acne want to know about squeezing spots, and the Acne Support Group gives very practical advice on this matter (www.stopspots.org). In summary, if it is a blackhead squeeze it gently (not using the fingernails) having washed the hands. Stop squeezing when nothing appears, and preferably before it starts to bleed. If the spot is red and angry but no pus is visible, it should not be squeezed. However, if pus is visible a similar technique to squeezing blackheads should be used – i.e. use gentle pressure with the fingers, and stop before it bleeds. A dab of antiseptic is a good idea afterwards.

Pregnancy

Many women notice changes in their skin and hair during the course of their monthly cycles as a result of the hormonal changes that take place. These hormonal changes occur due to the activity of hormones secreted by the ovaries, mainly oestrodial and progesterone. It is during the second half of the cycle, following ovulation when the progesterone level peaks, that women notice changes in the skin and sometimes exacerbation of an existing condition.

Most women notice an increase in skin pigmentation during pregnancy. Areas that are already pigmented become darker, in particular the nipples, areola, genital area and the midline of the abdominal wall. The pigmentation usually fades following delivery, but seldom to its previous level. The number and size of melanocytic naevi (moles) often increases. In a large proportion of women (about 70 per cent) chloasmal pigmentation develops during the second half of the pregnancy. This is characterized by irregular, sharply marginated areas of pigmentation that develop in a symmetrical pattern either on the forehead and temples or in the central part of the face. It usually fades following delivery.

Many women maintain that hair growth on the scalp is more vigorous during pregnancy but that it decreases after delivery of the baby, and this shedding of hair may result in noticeable post-partum alopecia (Winton and Lewis, 1982).

Ageing

From birth to old age, the skin gradually changes. The epidermis is thinner in old age due to the diminished mitotic activity of basal cells in the epidermis and the fact that the cells take longer to migrate to the stratum corneum. This contributes to the thin, shiny appearance of old skin (Franz and Gardner, 1994). Aged skin often has a greater number of pigment spots; although in general the numbers of melanocytes decreases there is an increase in specific areas which results in the pigment spots – especially on light-exposed skin. Hormonal changes means that there is less sebum secreted onto the skin surface, which explains why older skin tends to be very dry. Within the dermis, elastic fibres are lost and so the skin is less elastic. Collagen is also lost and this, combined with the redistribution of subcutaneous fat, causes sagging of the skin and the formation of folds (Ebbersole and Hess, 1998).

Many of the changes we tend to relate to old age are actually the result of (or are at the very least exacerbated by) accumulative ultraviolet damage from years of sun exposure. The importance of ultraviolet radiation in producing ageing is demonstrated by the contrast between exposed and covered skin. The face, neck and the backs of the hands always look much older than the trunk. These changes are much more dramatic in outdoor workers (Nicol and Fsenske, 1993).

A tan is part of the skin's defence against sun damage, but premature wrinkling and leathery looking skin are other symptoms of prolonged exposure to the sun. More sinister, however, is the link between over-exposure to the sun and the manifestation of sun-induced skin cancers. Skin cancer can be directly linked to sun exposure and damage, and whilst most skin cancers are easily treated, some, like malignant melanoma, can be deadly. Ultraviolet radiation is always present, although levels vary depending on the time of year. Even on cloudy days or in the shade, 75 per cent of the sun's rays still reach the earth (Lamana, 1996).

The only effective way of minimizing sun-induced skin ageing is by very careful avoidance of sunlight from birth. The genetic make-up of an individual determines where and to what extent age-related changes occur. Different individuals, even those with identical colouring, respond to similar exposure to sunlight with great variation, some looking old and wizened, others much younger. Protection from the sun is therefore important at all stages of life, since 'sun is to skin cancer what cigarettes are to lung cancer'.

Caring for the skin

Even skin that is termed 'normal' requires looking after, and the basic principles are the same whether the skin is that of a baby or octogenarian. Emollient therapy (the use of moisturizers) is the key. Basically, skin needs to be kept clean, moisturized and free from infection (Spencer, 1988). Although these principles are relevant to all age groups, meticulous skin care and in particular moisturizing is of special importance for the older person.

Bathing

Dry skin is caused by evaporation of water from the epidermis, which causes the skin to tighten and feel uncomfortable. The hot, dry conditions in hospital make this more likely. Moisturizing the skin can help to reduce trans-epidermal water loss by creating a surface film of lipid, which slows down the loss of water. This layer also helps to provide a protective barrier from the environment (Marks, 1997). Adding bath oil to the water will help to rehydrate the skin by increasing the oil-to-water ratio and so making the water greasy. For this reason it is important that older people are made aware that the bath will become very slippery when bath oil is used, and that they may need help to get out safely. Parents with small babies also need to be warned, as babies also become very slippery and it may be difficult to keep a tight hold of them. If a patient is unable to get into a bath, then bath oil can be added to the wash bowl. If the patient wishes to shower, there are a number of products available in moisturizing shower gel formulation. The soap substitutes discussed in the next section can be used as an alternative or in addition to the use of bath emollients.

Soap substitutes

Soap removes dirt and excess oil, but it also removes the skin's natural oils and therefore increases skin dehydration. If the skin is already dry, soap accentuates the problem and should therefore be avoided. There are a large number of soap substitutes available in the form of creams, lotions and ointments (e.g. aqueous cream, Wash E45™ and emulsifying ointment respectively), but there are no hard and fast rules about which one to choose. The best guide is the patient's preference and, as will be seen in the next section, creams, lotions and ointments all have different beneficial properties. Soap substitutes can either be used by massaging them gently onto each area of the body in turn and then rinsing them off or by putting an amount of the substitute on a flannel and gently rubbing the body as with normal soap.

Care must be taken not to over-wash the skin, as this will remove natural oils (such as sebum) as well as the commensal bacteria that live harmlessly on the skin and prevent the growth of potentially pathogenic bacteria.

Moisturizers

After washing, the skin needs to be carefully dried, preferably by patting – not by vigorous rubbing, which tends to damage delicate or dry skin and aggravate itchy skin. A moisturizer can then be applied. Moisturizers or emollients (different words for the same thing) are best applied immediately following a bath, as the skin is warm and at its most receptive. The resulting oily barrier will prevent further water loss (Heenan, 1996). Moisturizers come in three forms; creams, lotions and ointments. The general rule for moisturizers is the greasier they are, the better they are at rehydrating the skin.

[NB: It is easy to get confused over what a good moisturizer is. The word makes it sound as if water will moisturize, and this is not the case; water actually dries the skin. The word moisturizer refers to a substance's ability to retain the natural moisture of the skin and lubricate it with grease (Dawkes, 1997a).]

Creams are a mixture of oil and water. Under normal circumstances these two elements will not mix, so stabilizers are added. Creams rub into the skin easily without leaving the skin looking greasy, and this makes them popular with patients. They do have the disadvantage of needing to contain preservatives in order to prevent the cream becoming contaminated by bacteria or fungi. All preservatives can act as sensitizers and cause a contact allergic reaction. Experimentation using just small areas of skin will indicate whether someone is sensitive to the creams or not. If new products are being tried, it is best if a test area is left for 48 hours before applying the cream to the whole body in case of a delayed reaction. Creams are best used for chronic episodes or maintenance of the skin quality.

Lotions are liquid creams, and tend to have a cooling effect on the skin. They tend to be less effective at moisturizing than creams or ointments; however, they are a good choice for normal skin care although again they will contain preservatives.

Ointments are oil-based and contain very little water. Their main ingredient is usually white soft paraffin, which is semi-solid at room temperature but melts at around body temperature, making it easy to rub into the skin. As neither bacteria nor fungi can grow in this medium there is no need to add preservatives, so ointments are unlikely to cause an adverse reaction. They are very greasy to the touch, which means that they are messy to use. Ointments form a layer over the skin that prevents transepidermal water loss. This layer is more impenetrable than the layer created by a cream, and is therefore more effective. Other oils may be added to alter the smell or consistency of the ointment, as in emulsifying ointment (emulsifying wax 30 per cent, liquid paraffin 20 per cent, white soft paraffin 50 per cent). Ointments are best used during an acute or subacute episode where the skin has become very dry and inflamed, especially at night time, as they hydrate the skin well.

Applying moisturizers

The principle of applying moisturizers is very simple – start at the top and work down. Moisturizers, whatever their form, should be applied using downward strokes in the same direction that the hair follicles grow; this will prevent the problem of blocked hair follicles and the resulting folliculitis (inflamed or infected follicles that present as a small pustule). Patients are often worried about using too much grease, so it is important to stress that if properly applied you can never use too much moisturizer (Dawkes, 1997a).

When recommending moisturizers, there are many factors to be taken into consideration. How dry is the patient's skin? How much time a day does the patient have for treating the skin? Is the moisturizer for use in hospital or at home? What facilities does the patient have for doing laundry? Which moisturizer does the patient find most cosmetically acceptable? If possible, it is always best to use the greasiest moisturizer that the patient will tolerate. However, there can be problems with this. The moisturizers tend to soak into the clothes as well as the skin, and so can get onto soft furnishings and bed linen. The very greasy moisturizers can be difficult to wash out of some clothes, and the oil in some moisturizers can damage the rubber seal on washing machines. It is far better for a patient to select – and use – a less greasy moisturizer than not use one at all.

The scalp

Most people will at some time in their lives be affected by a dry scalp and in the majority of cases this will respond to a suitable shampoo, provided that it is used on alternate days at least. Most shampoos of this type contain a solution of coal tar (Polytar™ liquid, Alphosyl™ and T-Gel™ are common examples). Some people find the coal tar irritating and may prefer a milder shampoo. If the scalp remains excessively dry, it may be necessary to apply coconut oil at night. Coconut oil has a melting point close to that of body temperature, which means that if it is kept somewhere cool it is a solid but it will become a liquid once in contact with the skin. The most successful way to apply coconut

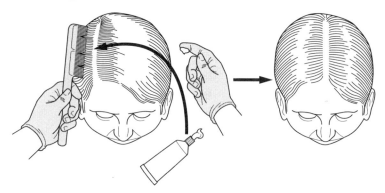

Figure 2.5 For treatment of scalp. 1. Hair is parted using comb; 2. Ointment rubbed in along exposed section of scalp; 3. Repeat, parting hair in different sections until complete scalp is covered.

oil is to part the hair and rub the oil into the scalp along the parting, then to part the next section of hair and repeat the process, continuing until the entire scalp has been treated (see Figure 2.5) (Dawkes, 1997b). The oil is then ideally left on the head over night and washed out in the morning, taking care to protect pillows with old pillowcases.

This method can be time consuming, but is the most effective way to get the treatment to the affected scalp. If possible it is better to teach a relative or friend to apply the oil, as it is difficult for patients to reach the back of their own head.

The differences between black and white skin

Black skin varies from white skin in that the epidermal cells contain more melanin. Melanin is produced by the melanocytes in the basal layer of the epidermis, and it is this that is responsible for the skin's colour and its ability to tan. The actual number of melanocytes is not greater in black skin, but they are more effective and produce more melanin. Whilst the basic function and structure of black skin is the same as white skin, there are certain differences that need to be considered.

Black skin does not react to exposure to sunlight by producing a tan, but it does show the same effects of sun over time as white skin – i.e. ageing and wrinkling. It is therefore equally important to educate Afro-Caribbean and Asian people about wearing a hat and T-shirt and applying a sunblock with high UVA and UVB protection factors.

If damaged either by trauma or disease, black skin often produces hyperpigmentation at the site of the healing lesion. This can cause considerable problems cosmetically, especially if a young person with acne has been treated successfully only to be left with hyperpigmented areas on their face. These areas will usually fade, although the individual will need considerable reassurance and support. Depigmentation can also occur as a result of atopic eczema; once again this will usually resolve with the correct use of topical steroids.

Black skin is more prone to developing keloids, probably because of a genetic predisposition. These abnormal scars are caused by an overgrowth of collagen in the skin, which arises in response to trauma; they are hard and smooth and can be domed, linear or irregular, all with claw-like projections. The most common sites for keloids are the ear lobes, shoulders, upper chest, neck, back and abdomen. All black patients should be asked about familial tendencies to keloids prior to elective surgery in order to minimize the risk of one occurring at the site of the incision.

In terms of day-to-day care of black skin, two factors are important. First, black skin tends to be much drier than white skin and will need more frequent moisturizing. Second, Afro-Caribbean men are more prone to developing in-grown hairs around the beard area following shaving. This is because the hair follicle is curved. The razor cuts the beard and leaves an obliquely pointed hair, which is more prone to re-entering the skin and thus causing an inflammatory reaction. Occasionally this may be misdiagnosed as acne.

Conclusion

Normal skin is a complex organ, and is not just a wrapping to keep our internal organs in the right place. It is capable of rapid regeneration and is responsible for many of the body's reactions to the environment, including protection, temperature control and providing us with sensory information. It gives non-verbal information about ourselves to others, and has a profound effect on psychological well-being. Like our other organs, it needs looking after if it is to continue to function to its full potential. We spend time and money on keeping fit so that organs like the heart will last a lifetime. If our skin is to do the same, it needs to be given similar attention.

Reflective activities

1. Give some further thought to how culture affects skin care and display of skin. Consider patients you have looked after, and how have you managed their cultural differences in terms of display, touch and privacy.
2. Think about what skin care is given to your patients and how much thought is given to it. Is there anything you might like to change?
3. Think about your own sunbathing habits. Discuss these with your colleagues and find out what their habits are. Gather information and posters to put together a display on the dangers of sun worshipping.

References

Black, P. A. (1995). Acne vulgaris. *Prof. Nurse*, **11(3)**, 181–3.
Brooker, C. (1998). *Human Structure and Function: Nursing Applications in Clinical Practice*, 2nd edn. CV Mosby Co.
Carroll, H. (2000). Oh, for perfect skin. *The Guardian*, **15 Jul**.
Cork, M. J. (1997). The importance of skin barrier function. *J. Dermatolog. Treatment*, **8(Suppl. 1)**, s7–s13.
Dawkes, K. (1997a). How to ... apply emollients effectively. *Br. J. Dermatol. Nursing*, **1(2)**, 8–9.
Dawkes, K. (1997b). How to ... treat scalp psoriasis. *Br. J. Dermatol. Nursing*, **1(1)**, 8–9.
Davies, H. (1997). *Introductory Immunobiology*. Chapman & Hall.
Ebbersole, P. and Hess, P. (1998). *Toward Health: Aging. Human Needs and Nursing Response*, 5th edn. CV Mosby Co.
Franz, R. A. and Gardner, S. (1994). Elderly skin care: principles of chronic wound care. *J. Gerontolog. Nursing*, **20(9)**, 35–44.
Heenan, A. (1996). Emollient applications for chronic skin problems. *Prof. Nurse*, **11(11)**, 743–8.
Holick, M. F., MacLaughlin, J. A. and Doppelt, S. H. (1981). Factors that influence the cutaneous photosynthesis of previtamin D. *Science*, **211**, 590–93.
Hunter, J. A. A., Savin, J. A. and Dahl, M. V. (1995). *Clinical Dermatology*, 2nd edn. Blackwell Science.
Lamanna, L. (1996). Be on the look out for skin cancer. *Am. J. Nursing*, **96(8)**, 16A, 16C–D.
Marks, R. (1997). How to measure the effects of emollients. *J. Dermatolog. Treatment*, **8(Suppl. 1)**, s15–s18.
Martini, F. (1998). *Foundation of Anatomy and Physiology*. Prentice Hall.
Morris, D. (1977). *Manwatching: A Field Guide to Human Behaviour*. Triad/Panther Books.
Morton, O. (1993). Here comes the sun. *Nursing Times*, **89(29)**, 52–4.
National Institute for Clinical Excellence. (2000). *Referral Practice: A Guide to Appropriate Referral from General to Specialist Services* (Version under pilot).

Neff, C. and Spray, M. (1996). *Introduction to Maternal and Child Health Nursing.* Lippincott.

Nicol, N. H. and Fsenske, N. A. (1993). Photodamage: cause, clinical manifestations and prevention. *Dermatol. Nursing*, **5(4)**, 263–77.

Novotny, J. (1989). Adolescents, acne, and other side effects of accutane. *Ped. Nursing*, **15(3)**, 247–8.

Perkins, P. (1993). Prevention through education: a pilot study on skin cancer education in primary schools. *Child Health*, **Oct/Nov**, 117–22.

Rook, A., Wilkinson, D. S. and Ebling, A. (1979). The *Textbook of Dermatology*. Blackwell Scientific.

Shuster, S. (1981). Dermatological dog fights: confessions of a middle-aged academic. *World Med.*, **4 Apr**, 77–87.

Spencer, T. S. (1988). Dry skin and skin moisturisers. *Clin. Dermatol.*, **6(3)**, 24–8.

Spindler, J. R. and Data, J. L. (1992). Female androgenic alopecia: a review. *Dermatol. Nursing*, **4(2)**, 93–9.

Walsh, M., Crumbie, A. and Reveley, S. (2001). *Nurse Practitioners: clinical skills and professional issues*. Butterworth-Heinemann, Oxford.

Winton, G. B. and Lewis, C. W. (1982). Dermatoses of pregnancy. *J. Am. Acad. Dermatol.*, **6**, 977–8.

3
Abnormal skin: how it functions and how to look after it

Fiona Pringle and Rebecca Penzer

Introduction

When the skin fails it can do so, broadly speaking, in one of three ways. It may stop functioning normally because of:

1. An internal factor, usually a systemic disease
2. An external factor such as an environmental influence (e.g. moisture caused by incontinence)
3. A dermatological condition (i.e. where the primary focus of the disease is the skin, rather than the skin altering due to other factors).

This chapter explores all three of the above within the context of nursing care and the experiences that patients have.

Skin changes due to a systemic disease

When a person's general health is impaired, the skin can provide important signs of this fact. For example, pallor denotes fewer red blood cells in the skin because of anaemia or peripheral vasoconstriction, and the first sign of liver disease may be jaundice noted in the skin. Fever may be noted by the warmth of the skin, and changes in skin texture, moisture, pigmentation and hair distribution all give clues about electrolyte, endocrine and nutritional balance. This section explores these issues by focusing on key symptoms that a nurse can identify through observing the skin. It is not possible to mention all the potential skin changes that can take place in systemic disease; however, this section highlights the most common ones.

Changes in pigmentation

Jaundice is the name of the yellow colour given to the skin by the bile pigment bilirubin. It occurs when the liver is unable to break down and excrete bilirubin, thus leading to its build-up in the skin. The whites of the eyes can also turn yellow. It indicates an advanced stage of liver failure.

Hyperpigmentation (increased level of pigment in the skin) is a common symptom of several systemic diseases. It is caused by an increase in the amount of melanin in the epidermis, which happens in response to the pituitary producing melanocyte-stimulating hormone (MSH). In healthy adults the pituitary does not secrete MSH except in pregnant women (explaining the changes in pigment associated with pregnancy; see Chapter 2). However, the pituitary does produce MSH in a number of systemic diseases, causing hyperpigmentation. There is as yet no satisfactory explanation as to why the body does this, as it does not seem to have any positive benefit for the individual. Diseases where hyperpigmentation occurs include liver disease and hyperthyroidism.

Overproduction of adrenocorticotrophic hormone (ACTH) in both Addison's disease and Cushing's syndrome will also produce hyperpigmentation. This is because melanocyte-stimulating hormone is very similar in structure to ACTH, and therefore has the similar effect of producing an increase in pigment.

The nursing care for people with pigmentation changes will depend on the systemic disease they are suffering from. The changes are useful indicators, and can be used as part of the assessment process. Many patients will feel embarrassed about their skin changing colour, and may well be alarmed by it. Nurses must be ready to explain why the changes have happened and to offer psychological support as necessary. It is unlikely for an individual's colour to return to normal until the underlying cause of the systemic disease is treated, and this is not always possible.

Circulatory system

Changes in the circulatory system in response to systemic disease are wide ranging and numerous. Many of these changes can lead to an alteration in the skin's appearance or, more dramatically, the skin breaking down.

Cyanosis

Cellular hypoxia is indicated by the bluish hue of cyanosis, which is easily observed in the nail beds, lips and mucous membranes. Black skin usually assumes a greyish tone if cyanosed. It should be remembered that cyanosis occurs when more than 5 g/dl of haemoglobin is in the reduced state (i.e. not carrying oxygen).

Therefore cyanosis is more likely to be seen in someone with polycythaemia than in someone who is anaemic.

Inflammation

Inflammation occurs as the body's response to physical or chemical injury. There are five key features of the acute inflammatory response:

1. Redness (otherwise known as erythema) as the blood vessels dilate
2. Heat (otherwise known as hyperaemia) as the blood flow increases in that area
3. Swelling as fluid exudes from blood vessels
4. Pain due to chemical and pressure stimulation of the nerve endings
5. Loss of function, especially near to a joint.

Surgical or accidental trauma will both produce this inflammatory reaction; in these circumstances it is a normal and necessary part of skin repair. However, if the skin continues to be hot and red beyond 3 days after the trauma it is likely that there is some sort of bacterial infection. Although this may be accompanied by a pyrexia, observing the skin remains a useful way of monitoring postoperative infections.

Erythema and hyperaemia (without the rest of the inflammatory process) accompany many dermatological conditions, and these will be discussed later on in this chapter.

Adverse drug reactions are another cause of erythema. The most common drugs to cause problems are antibiotics (especially Ampicillin), sulphonamides and barbiturates.

Ulceration

When the epidermis is lost as a result of blistering, necrosis or trauma, a circumscribed, depressed, moist area appears. An erosion is an area of missing epidermis that extends no lower than the basal cell layer. Erosions heal without scarring.

An ulcer results when the entire epidermis is absent. Destruction of full-thickness epidermis and papillary dermis causes a superficial ulcer. Destruction down to the mid- or lower dermis causes a deep ulcer, which, if it heals, will leave a scar. Healing will be delayed because of poor circulation to the area. Poor circulation may be as a result of impaired venous or arterial blood flow, or because of pressure exerted on the area.

It is often difficult to determine the original cause of the ulceration, but information can be gained by noting the location and size of the ulcer or erosion and by examining other lesions that might be present. Nodules, plaques, varicose veins or excoriations that are nearby may be related to the cause of the ulcer. An ulcer may have a characteristic border, base or discharge. Taking a detailed patient history may reveal some trauma that resulted in an injury that would not heal and became ulcerated. Further information on ulcers is given in the section on wound assessment and care (see p. 58).

Malignancies

Malignancies that affect the skin can be divided into three groups:

1. Skin cancers
2. Changes in the skin owing to malignancy elsewhere
3. Tumours that metastasize to the skin.

As this section concerns the changes that occur to the skin because of systemic disease, skin cancers *per se* will not be considered here. For further information, see the section that looks at skin changes caused by the environment.

Changes in the skin due to systemic malignancies

There are a whole host of potential symptoms related to skin changes in people with systemic malignancies. The most common signs are pruritus, pallor due to anaemia, and pigment changes due to increased levels of melanin produced by cancer cells. Pruritus is most common in lymphoma, leukaemia, carcinoma and sarcoma; in Hodgkin's disease up to 25 per cent of sufferers experience pruritus at some point (Dangel, 1986). In general, suspicions should be aroused by any sudden changes in the appearance of the skin when there are no other explanations. Some specific signs to look out for are:

- Warty, hyperpigmented thickening in the skin of the axillae and groins (acanthosis nigricans), which is most commonly associated with an adenocarcinoma of the gastrointestinal tract. Note that this symptom is very commonly found in the obese, where it is unrelated to systemic problems.
- 'Fish-scale' skin (icthyosis), where the skin becomes very dry and there is widespread scaly dryness. Icthyosis is only associated with malignancy (especially lymphoma) when it develops suddenly in adult life.

- Bullous pemphigoid, which may be associated with internal malignancy.
- A sudden profuse development of seborrhoeic warts, known as the sign of Leser Trelat
- A sudden profuse growth of vellus hair over the face and body, which is a rare sign of malignancy.

Leukaemia often presents with purpura (a phenomena where red blood cells are forced out into the skin, making small red lesions that do not blanch with pressure), bruising, and bleeding from the gums. Bone marrow transplants, a treatment for leukaemia, can have an impact on the skin (as well as the liver and gut) if the transplant is rejected. In graft-versus-host reactions, the first signs that rejection is occurring are usually seen in the skin 2–3 weeks after transplantation. These signs include a measle-like eruption followed by erythema of the hands and feet.

Malignancies that metastasize to the skin

The most common malignant tumours that metastasize to the skin are renal, ovarian, gastrointestinal, breast and bronchial tumours. The metastases present initially as nondescript pink nodules, usually occurring on the scalp or the front of the abdomen. If left untreated they can ulcerate. Ovarian or gastrointestinal carcinomas can metastasize to an umbilical nodule known as Sister Joseph's nodule. Lymphatic extension of carcinoma of the skin can produce inflammation that looks similar to cellulitis.

Nursing care usually involves disease and symptom management. The strategies used to manage dry skin and itch (see Chapter 2) are most useful. Appropriate psychological support is vital to help patients cope with any sort of malignancy.

Pruritus

The symptom of itch accompanies many of the systemic changes highlighted above and most of the skin diseases discussed later in this chapter, and could therefore be appropriately discussed in either section. It seems true to say, however, that if the skin is involved in any way there is the potential for the symptom of itch to be present.

The management, description and aetiology of itch has challenged healthcare professionals for centuries. There is little doubt that this unpleasant sensation is experienced by many patients; however, it has always been difficult to ascertain to what extent the sensation is physiological or psychological in origin. After all, if any of us were to sit quietly and think about our skin for a few minutes, almost without fail we would feel an itch somewhere!

Itch can be described as an unpleasant sensation that leads to scratching, and although this description is not perfect it remains the one most commonly used (Savin, 1995). The scratch response occurs without thinking, and has evolved as a way of removing potentially harmful substances from the skin (Hagermark and Wahlgren, 1992). However, itch can occur when there is nothing harmful in contact with the skin, and the scratching itself can cause damage rather than prevent it. Much is still unknown about the neurophysiology of itch; it was thought that itch was a low-grade level of pain, but this theory has now been rejected. Pain and itch have been shown to be different for a number of reasons: they can both be felt at the same time; itch cannot be experienced if the epidermis is removed whereas pain can; and they elicit different responses from the sufferer – itching leads to scratching, and pain to withdrawal (Wahlgren, 1992).

The reason that pain and itch have been associated in the past is because it is believed that they are both transmitted by unmyelinated C-fibres. However, it is thought that the receptors for itch found in the epidermis may be specially developed to pick up information about itch, although this has not yet been proved (Bernhard, 1991). Because the nerve endings for itch are found only in the epidermis, itch is not felt if the epidermis is removed.

Although the sensation of itch is transmitted through the C-fibres, there are other substances responsible for the production of the itch sensation. Histamine is the classic itch mediator, but it by no means functions alone. Certain proteolytic enzymes and peptides act as histamine releasers, prostaglandins seem to reduce the threshold for histamine-induced itch, and serotonin itself seems to induce itch (Denman, 1986).

The psychological impact of itch can be enormous, with the physical sensation of itch being akin to torture for some patients. Patients describe a feeling of things crawling across or, worse still, under their skin, and often scratch to the point where they break the skin. Pain is seen as preferable to itch by some. Although scratching provides some temporary relief, it worsens itchy sensations and the 'itch–scratch' cycle can ensue (Bridgett, 1996). The act of scratching also leads to difficulties in social situations, as scratching is seen as socially unacceptable because of the connotations of dirtiness or infestation. The restlessness of scratching at night may not keep the sufferer awake, but is likely to disturb the sleep of a partner.

There is little clear evidence about the impact of psychological status on the experience of itch, although it is thought that this does have a part to play. Research into using habit reversal as a way of controlling scratching has shown some beneficial results (Noren and Melin, 1989). The fact that people itch more at night than during the day may be due in part to the fact that they have no distractions. Frustratingly, some people itch with no apparent cause; in these situations the only option for the sufferer is to learn how to manage the symptoms.

Therefore, although itching is often not seen as an important symptom, it can have major affects on quality of life. Nursing care should help to manage the symptoms, and is based on the following principles:

• Keeping the environment as cool and as dust-free as possible
• Wearing loose cotton clothing
• Making sure that the skin is well moisturized
• Occluding the skin with the techniques discussed in Chapter 4 to prevent scratching and the itch–scratch cycle
• Avoiding contact with substances that are known to act as sensitizers
• Taking the symptom seriously, as many patients feel that the symptom of itch is at best misunderstood and at worst ignored.

Bridgett (1996) also advocates keeping a positive approach and encouraging habit reversal, as much scratching is done without thinking.

Skin changes in relation to the environment

This section relates how the environment can impact on the skin. The term 'environment' is taken in its broadest sense, and includes the negative impact that the sun, external trauma and certain substances have on the skin.

Skin cancers

Cancers of the skin can be divided into two groups, those that are malignant and those that are benign. In both of these groups there are a number of different cancers, which are named according to the structure of the skin involved (Table 3.1). A typology of skin cancers is potentially complex and therefore, for the purpose of

Table 3.1 Commonly occurring cancers of the skin

Structure of the skin	Dysplastic/malignant	Benign
Epidermis	Actinic (solar) keratoses	Seborrhoeic keratoses
	Squamous cell carcinoma	Skin tags
	Basal cell carcinoma	Epidermal cysts
Melanocytes	Malignant melanoma	Freckle/lentigo
Dermis	Sarcomas	Dermatofibroma
		Vascular tumours
Lymph cells	Mycosis fungoides	

this section, the only the most commonly occurring cancers will be noted.

The most important elements of nursing care when considering skin tumours are support and education. There has been a huge increase in awareness of skin cancers and consequently the public needs to have clear advice from healthcare professionals. Descriptions of the benign lesions are given so that a distinction between these and malignant lesions can be made. Although these lesions may be of concern cosmetically, they do not threaten health.

Benign lesions

Seborrhoeic keratoses (also known as seborrhoeic warts) are very common in the older population, and present as flat-topped areas of skin that look as though they have been stuck onto the skin. They vary in shade from pale to dark, and generally their surface is not smooth and it has a number of indentations and irregularities on it. There may be just one or two of seborrhoeic keratoses present, but often they are numerous and scattered, usually over the head, neck, the back of the hands and forearms, and the trunk.

Skin tags look similar to seborrhoeic keratoses but form pedunculated lesions – i.e. they hang off the surface of the skin like a tag. Both skin tags and seborrhoeic keratoses can be removed using curettage and cautery (scraping away with a sharp 'spoon' and then applying heat to stem the bleeding). Liquid nitrogen may be used to 'freeze' the smaller lesions in a process known as cryotherapy.

Epidermal cysts are round, dome-like swellings of the skin, often with a central punctum (hole) through which the contents (a 'cheesy' substance) can be squeezed. Larger epidermal cysts may follow on from acne, whereas the smaller cysts (known as milia) may occur after trauma, although they are also known to be familial and develop spontaneously. Both types of cyst can be removed, the smaller ones using a sterile needle and the larger by incision under local anaesthetic. *NB*: Milia in newborn babies should not be removed, as they will resolve spontaneously (see Chapter 2).

Freckles are areas of skin where the melanocytes are particularly sensitive to UV radiation. They are most common in fair-skinned people.

Lentigines are permanent flat areas of skin that are composed of increased numbers of melanocytes.

Dermatofibromas are again very common, especially in women, and consist of fibrous tissue and some blood vessels. They may be pigmented or the colour of normal skin, and are most easily identified through touch; they feel as though there is a small, hard object (like a grain of uncooked rice) under the skin. They can be excised if they cause cosmetic concerns.

Vascular tumours (angiomas) consist of unusual blood vessels within the epidermis. Some of these present in newborns and others in adults. Commonly the latter are seen as deep red, slightly raised papules, known as Campbell de Morgan spots.

Pre-malignant or malignant lesions

These are the lesions that give greater concern in terms of their risk to health. Although some skin cancers may be due to other external factors (e.g. contact with carcinogenic compounds), the vast majority are due to exposure to the sun.

Actinic keratoses are pre-malignant lesions (Basler, 1991). They present as red, scaly patches on sun-exposed sites such as the dorsa of the hands and bald patches on the scalp. In people who have had excessive sun exposure there may be hundreds of these lesions. Although the malignant potential is small, they should usually be treated using liquid nitrogen.

Squamous cell carcinomas can either be invasive or non-invasive. The non-invasive type has low malignant potential and is known as Bowen's disease. The usual presentation is a single patch of red, scaly skin in a sun-exposed site; when the scale is removed, the patch left has a glistening red surface. Treatment is with liquid nitrogen or curettage. Invasive squamous cell carcinoma is much more serious, as it can metastasize to local lymph nodes and beyond. Presentation may involve ulcers, rapidly growing polypoid masses and keratotic lumps. A squamous cell carcinoma may be surrounded by actinic keratoses. Again, sun-exposed sites in the elderly are where squamous cell carcinomas are most commonly seen; the lips and mouth might be involved, those who smoke being particularly at risk.

Basal cell carcinomas (often called rodent ulcers) are the most common skin cancer. They usually occur on the face, although other areas are sometimes affected. A basal cell carcinoma starts off as a nodule, which gradually spreads out, leaving a depression in the middle of the lesion and the classic appearance of a 'rolled edge'. They are often translucent in colour, and may have very fine blood vessels known as telangiectasia running across the surface. These bleed very easily. Although basal cell carcinomas rarely metastasize they can be destructive locally, and need to be removed through excision, curettage or liquid nitrogen.

Of the malignant melanomas, the most common type seen in the United Kingdom is known as the superficial spreading melanoma, which affects a much younger population than squamous or basal cell carcinoma. They can occur anywhere on the body, and present as a brown/black lesion with an irregular border and a tendency to itch or cause discomfort. The severity of a malignant melanoma is measured by the depth that it has penetrated into the skin tissues. Surgical removal is the treatment of choice.

Sarcomas are cancers of connective tissue, and may arise in the skin. They present initially as nodules that do not clear up and grow relatively slowly. Of particular interest is Kaposi's sarcoma, which starts as pigmented purplish plaques on the legs and then progresses over the body. When Kaposi's sarcoma is seen in AIDS patients, it presents as multiple nodules.

Mycosis fungoides is a disease in which the T lymphocytes develop in an aberrant way. This results in a number of skin changes, although generally these are very slow and develop over several years. They will initially appear as well-circumscribed red, scaly areas, which are easy to confuse with psoriasis. As the disease progresses these can ulcerate. Treatment may involve radiotherapy or chemotherapy.

Nursing care

Successfully diagnosing skin cancer is usually a medical role, but it is vital that nurses remain aware of the wide range of skin cancers that exist and are particularly vigilant about those that can endanger life. Frequently there is a need to rely on taking a skin biopsy to determine the exact nature of a skin cancer. This way, cell changes can be viewed and a diagnosis made.

From a nursing perspective, the hardest part of identifying a skin cancer is deciding whether a mole is purely innocent or whether it is a malignant melanoma. Squamous and basal cell carcinomas have some unique features (see Table 3.1) that aid diagnosis. The ABCD rule (Somma and Glassman, 1991) is an aid in differentiating between an innocent mole and a malignant melanoma:

A – Asymmetry. A malignant melanoma is asymmetrical, where as a mole will look the same on one side as the other.
B – Borders. The borders of a malignant melanoma are irregular and may be blurred, whereas a mole has a definite regular outline.
C – Colour. A malignant melanoma is not evenly coloured and will range from brown to black with possible red and blue hues; a mole is evenly coloured.
D – Diameter. A malignant melanoma is usually greater than 6 mm in diameter, whereas moles are usually less than this. A sudden increase in size is cause for concern.

Exposure to UV radiation is the most common cause of any of the skin cancers. The fashion for a tan means that people choose risky behaviours (van der Weyden, 1994) to ensure that they get a 'healthy' golden glow. This risky behaviour includes the short, sharp exposures to the sun now available to increasing numbers of the population through cheap travel abroad. Nurses can help by providing clear guidance that does not prohibit some sun exposure but minimizes the damage it can cause. Nicole and Fenske (1993) highlight seven key messages that need to be transmitted:

1. Wear protective clothing, including a hat and close-weave long-sleeved T-shirt
2. Use a sunscreen of at least SPF 15 (and three stars)
3. Avoid sun exposure in the heat of the day (11 am–3 pm)
4. Be aware of photosensitizing chemicals (e.g. perfume and hairspray) and medications (e.g. tetracyclines and frusemide)
5. Be aware of the side effects of intentional sun exposure
6. Avoid reflective surfaces (e.g. sand, snow, concrete)
7. Avoid tanning machines.

As well as education, the nurse also has a very strong role to play in support following diagnosis. Being able to give clear information about what to expect, as well as providing psychological support, is vital.

Wounds

Wounds are usually caused by an external factor, either surgical or traumatic. Even leg ulcers are often started by some small traumatic injury that does not heal properly, which is why they are discussed in this section.

Wound care has traditionally been an area of nursing surrounded by mystique and unsubstantiated practice (e.g. blowing oxygen onto wounds and spreading egg white over them). However, it is an area of practice where nurses are developing expertise beyond that of their medical colleagues, most especially in chronic wound care.

Categorizing wounds as chronic or acute is a useful way to understand the processes that are involved. Acute wounds occur as a result of trauma or surgery, whereas chronic wounds are long-standing in nature, e.g. pressure sores, leg ulcers and fungating lesions (Flanagan, 1994). Acute wounds may become chronic if they do not heal within what would be considered a normal timeframe.

Most acute wounds heal by primary intention. The opposing sides of an acute wound are normally held together with stitches, which allows healing to occur through all the layers of muscle and skin (Figure 3.1a). Most chronic wounds heal by secondary intention, which occurs when the sides of the wound are not held together and so healing has to occur from the wound bed (Figure 3.1b). Generally, managing chronic wounds is more complex and involved than managing acute wounds.

The aim here is to cover four key issues with relation to wound care:

1. Assessment
2. Cleansing
3. Dressing choice
4. Bandaging.

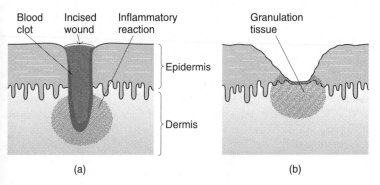

Figure 3.1 Wound healing: (a) by primary intention; (b) by secondary intention.

Special attention will be given to the care of leg ulcers, as these are good examples of chronic wounds:

Assessment

Assessment of wounds requires a holistic approach, i.e. wounds should not be considered in isolation but must be viewed within the context of the individual's general health and social circumstances. Thus as well as gathering data regarding the wound itself, its position on the body, its depth, the appearance of the wound bed and the surrounding skin (Benbow, 1995), questions must be asked about the patient's background social as well as medical history.

There are a number of different tools to help with wound assessment. The Wound Care Society has published a useful one (see Figure 3.2) that guides the nurse through the process of wound assessment (Flanagan, 1994). It includes a box labelled 'non-compliance', and indeed a problem in chronic wound care is that of patients not adhering to their dressing regime. However, this often requires exploring rather than labelling patients 'non-compliant', as there are frequently understandable reasons why they are not adhering to treatment regimes. These factors need to be identified and tackled. Such factors might include poorly managed pain, dressings that limit mobility or the ability to put a shoe on, or lack of motivation and the feeling that nothing will ever improve. (See Chapter 5 for a discussion of compliance and concordance.)

When assessing any sort of chronic wounds, all the above factors need to be taken into account. There are, however, additional factors that will impact upon the way that a leg ulcer is managed, and these are primarily because of the differing aetiology of leg ulcers.

Assessing a leg ulcer

Ulcers can be caused either by venous or arterial insufficiency (and occasionally a mixture of the two). Arterial insufficiency includes atherosclerosis, in which the arteries are hardened and narrowed so that arterial blood flow is reduced. This might be caused by hypertension or smoking, and means that the amount of oxygenated blood reaching the lower limbs is decreased. Venous insufficiency is due to the valves in the veins working less efficiently so that deoxygenated blood tends to 'pool' in the lower extremities. A family history of venous disease, having a job that involves standing still (particularly in a warm environment) and obesity all predispose an individual to venous disease.

Initial assessment

Names

Patient	Age

GP name

Describe the wound

Type of wound

Location of wound

Wound dimensions

Max length [   ] cm/mm (Delete as appropriate)

Max width [   ] cm/mm (Delete as appropriate)

Depth [   ] cm/mm (Delete as appropriate)

Length of time wound present [   ] days/weeks/months/years (Delete as appropriate)

Risk assessment

Pressure sore risk assessment scale used [   ]   Score [   ]

Doppler reading = $\dfrac{\text{Ankle pressure}}{\text{Arm pressure}}$ [   ] mm/Hg   Index [   ]

Condition of skin [   ] Good/intact   [   ] Fair/red areas*   [   ] Poor/breaks*

*Describe in more detail together with action taken

Factors that may delay healing

Diabetes	[ ]	Medications	[ ]
Anaemia	[ ]	Allergies	[ ]
Immobility	[ ]	Non-compliance	[ ]
Poor nutritional status	[ ]	Others	[ ]

Referral requested   Date

Clinical nurse specialist	[ ]
Dermatologist	[ ]
Vascular surgeon	[ ]
Dietitian	[ ]
Chiropodist	[ ]
Others	[ ]

Figure 3.2 Wound care assessment tool. (Reproduced with kind permission from Wound Care Society, Huntingdon)

Ongoing assessment

Date of dressing change										
Wound dimensions										
Max length (cm/mm)										
Max width (cm/mm)										
Depth (cm/mm)										
Are dimensions . . .										
Increasing?										
Decreasing?										
Static?										
Wound bed (approx. %cover)										
Necrotic (black)										
Slough (yellow)										
Granulating (red)										
Epithelialising (pink)										
Exudate levels										
High*										
Moderate										
Low										
Amount increasing*										
Amount decreasing										
*May indicate wound infection										
Wound margin/surrounding skin										
Macerated*										
Oedematous										
Erythema*										
Eczema										
Fragile*										
Dry/scaling										
Healthy/intact										
*May indicate wound infection										
Pain*										
Continuous										
At specific times										
At dressing change										
None										
*May indicate wound infection										
In addition, suspect wound infection if . . .										
Granulation tissue bleeds easily										
Fragile bridging of epithelium occurs										
Odour increases										
Healing is slower than expected										
Wound breakdown										
Action taken										
Swab sent										
Results obtained										
Treatment objective(s)										
Debridement										
Absorption										
Hydration										
Protection										
Documentation (7–10 day intervals) — tick when done										
Trace wound circumference										
Photograph										
Evaluate pressure risk-assessment score										
Signature/initial										

It is vital that the nature of the ulcer is determined, as this will dictate the right treatment. Four key strategies need to be employed for this assessment:

1. Detection of a pulse in the foot suggests that arterial flow is still present and that the ulcer is therefore venous. This can be done by feeling for a pedal pulse on the dorsum of the foot, although this can sometimes be difficult, especially if there is a lot of oedema present. A Doppler reading is much more accurate and reliable. A Doppler is a small ultrasonic probe that can be moved over the dorsum of the foot to pick up blood-flow sounds. To identify whether the ulcer is arterial or venous, the systolic blood pressure reading in the arm is measured and then, using the Doppler, the blood pressure in the foot is measured (Rich, 2001). If the systolic reading in the leg is the same or greater than that in the arm the ulcer is venous. Often a calculation is made to give the ankle pressure index (API), which expresses the two blood pressure readings as a ratio: systolic pressure in the leg/systolic pressure in the arm. For example, if the systolic pressure in the arm is 120 and the systolic pressure in the leg is 130, the ankle pressure index is 1.08. Therefore a quick way to describe whether an ulcer is venous or arterial is to express the API – if it is greater or equal to 1 the ulcer is venous; if it is less than 1 the ulcer is arterial. Specialist training is required to be able to use a Doppler machine accurately.
2. Observation of the ulcer itself and the surrounding skin helps to determine the nature of the ulceration.

   • Venous ulcers can be almost any size from very small to being circumferential around a lower limb; however, they usually have a well-defined flat edge and tend to be present around the medial and lateral malleoli. Venous disease is often accompanied by tortuous veins, atrophy blanche (white patches caused by necrosis of the skin due to thrombosis in the iliac veins) and varicose eczema (which is red, scaly and itchy, and is caused by a build-up of metabolic waste products in the tissues). Oedema is also common, as the 'pooling' of fluid in the lower legs (venous hypertension) causes swelling.
   • Arterial ulcers have a more punched-out look and tend to be deeper. They occur on the shin, heel, dorsum of the foot and the toes, and the surrounding skin tends to be pale, scaly and cool. There is a reduction in the amount of hair on the legs, and the toenails are thickened.

3. Asking the patient how the ulcer feels will also provide some vital clues as to its nature, as well as helping with deciding the

most appropriate plan of care. Pain is a useful distinguishing factor as, although both types of ulcers are associated with pain, the pain as described by patients is very different. Venous ulcers can be very painful, although this is not usually related to the size; however, pain is usually decreased by elevation and is at its worse during or just after dressing changes. Arterial ulcers are much more painful on elevation, and patients will often get relief by dangling their foot over the edge of the bed. This is because when the leg is dangling, arterial flow is aided by gravity.

4. Recording the assessment process is vital for monitoring healing. Photography provides the most easily accessible visual record, but the photographs must be of good quality and taken with a scale reference next to the ulcer. Tracing is very helpful for monitoring size reduction, but the tracing must be marked to indicate which way up it goes so that on referring back to it the reference is accurate. From an infection control point of view, if tracings are to be stored in the notes care must be taken to ensure that the part of the tracing that has come into contact with the wound is discarded or cleaned. Measuring is perhaps the least satisfactory method of recording the ulcer, but if careful note is made of where the measurements are taken from it does provide some idea about the size. Clear written descriptions about the colour of the wound bed, the presence of any exudate, the state of the surrounding skin and how it feels to the patient, must all be made.

Further information about the evidence available for the assessment and treatment of venous ulcers is available in a Technical Report from the Royal College of Nursing Institute (Cullum *et al.*, 1998).

Cleansing

Methods for cleansing wounds have been subject to controversy, and often practice has been based upon ritualistic behaviour. The research in this field does indicate, however, that certain strategies will ensure safe practice. These will be discussed here, but it is important to remember that patients need to be assessed as individuals and care planned accordingly. For example, a patient who is severely immunocompromised may require a different approach.

The purpose of cleansing a wound is two-fold. Cleansing promotes the removal of loose wound and dressing debris and allows debridement of adherent necrotic or sloughing material

(Fletcher, 1997). In the past nurses have tended to over-clean wounds, using overly astringent cleaning agents. The drawbacks of over-cleaning include the removal of healthy growing tissue, excessive removal of exudate that might be promoting healing (Fletcher, 1997), a greater chance of cross-infection as the wound is exposed, and increased patient discomfort. The aim here is therefore to clarify what is actually necessary for the cleansing of both acute and chronic wounds.

Hollinworth and Kingston (1998), in a review of the literature on wound cleansing, suggest that in general a clean rather than aseptic approach is appropriate in most cases. Of utmost import- ance in the prevention of infection is effective hand washing on the part of the nurse, even if gloves are used. Gloves should be used but do not need to be sterile, and they advocate that the use of tap water for cleaning wounds is safe for most patients. Allowing patients with leg ulcers to soak their legs in a bucket of water is an effective way of removing debris. Oliver (1997) sug- gests that bathing for post-surgical patients is subject to greater debate, however; in some people and for some wounds closure to bacteria may occur within 6 hours of surgery, whereas for others it is likely to take more than 24 hours. Dealey (1994) states that primary wounds are usually closed 48 hours post-surgery and are therefore impervious to bacteria. Clearly individual assessment is needed, but bathing should be possible for most people within 2 days of surgery.

The concerns about using tap water centre on the existence of bacteria in the water. Whilst drinking water in Britain has very low levels of bacteria (Hollinworth and Kingston, 1998), if there are concerns about using water (either due to its lack of cleanli- ness or the fact that the patient is immunocompromised) other options should be used. The evidence regarding the use of anti- septics for wound cleaning is again controversial. There is no compelling evidence to say that antiseptics are better than normal saline (Oliver, 1997) and, in the absence of better evidence, normal saline is less potentially damaging than antiseptics.

When cleansing a wound, a balance must be struck between removing (debriding) tissue that will prevent wound healing and being overzealous with cleaning to the extent that healthy growing cells are removed. Thomlinson (1987) demonstrated that swabbing not only had the potential for leaving foreign bodies in the wound, but also distributed any bacteria from one area to another. Therefore, as a general rule:

• Wounds that have a healthy red base to them and pink epithe- lializing edges should be cleansed very gently or left alone and redressed; they should not be cleaned by dragging a swab soaked in saline across the wound, but rather by gentle irrigation using a syringe.

- Wounds with a slightly sloughy base to them will benefit from a leg jacuzzi, where the bubbles serve to clean the wound (Bergstrom *et al.*, 1994). If no leg jacuzzi is available, a bucket of water to soak the legs is helpful.

- Very sloughy or necrotic tissue will need to be removed. The former may be done using a de-sloughing agent such as Intrasite™, and the latter may require manual debridement using a scalpel (this should be done with great care as it is possible to cut through tendons, especially around the ankle; it is usually undertaken by a doctor). Increasingly, biosurgical techniques are being employed, where sterile maggots are introduced to the wound to eat away the dead tissue. Maggots will not eat healthy tissue, and therefore make excellent debriders (Thomas *et al.*, 1997).

Whatever wound cleanser is used, it is important that it is warm (around body temperature). Exposing healing wounds to cooler temperatures slows down the mitotic activity within the wound and therefore the speed at which it heals (Lock, 1980).

The presence of necrosis and slough do not necessarily indicate a clinical infection. The normal signs of a wound infection are erythema, swelling, pain and odour. Pseudomonas, for example, has a particularly distinctive 'eggy' smell and produces bright green exudate. If infection is suspected, a swab dampened with saline should be rolled across the wound bed and then put into a transport medium. A positive result along with clinical signs of infection will indicate that oral antibiotics are needed; topical antibiotics are rarely used because of the possibility of sensitization (Cooper and Lawrence, 1996).

Dressing choice

Choosing the appropriate dressing for a wound is a potential minefield. There are so many options that it sometimes seems baffling. Not only does the appropriate primary dressing (i.e. the one that goes next to and interacts with the wound) have to be chosen, but also the secondary dressings and bandages. There are no foolproof answers, but it is possible to outline some principles that help in the decision-making process:

- The wound must remain moist without being soggy; if a wound is too soggy the surrounding skin is in danger of becoming macerated and breaking down. Excess moisture is likely to cause frequent strikethrough, which may lead to infection.

- The wound must remain warm without being too warm, as this may encourage unwanted bacterial growth.
- The surrounding skin must be cared for meticulously, as it will be prone to breaking down.
- The wound bed should be pink/red and the edges healthy if healing is to occur.

When choosing a dressing, it helps to consider each of the above points in turn.

Exudate

If the wound is exuding, a dressing must absorb the exudate. The alginate (e.g. Sorbsan™) and foam (e.g. Lyfoam™ and Allevyn™) dressings are most effective for this. There are now alginate products that are specially designed for heavily exuding wounds. Lightly exuding wounds can often be managed with hydrocolloid dressings (e.g. Granuflex™) or a non-adherent dry dressing. The beauty of all of these dressings is that they are designed to interact with the wound bed in such a way as to minimize trauma on removal of the dressing. Alginates dissolve into a harmless soft mass that can be washed away (although it does not have to be), and the foams have surfaces that prevent them from sticking to the wound. Hydrocolloids 'dissolve' on contact with wound exudate and come away easily.

Dressing changes

Dressing changes should be kept to a minimum, and dressings should not be changed ritualistically. However, when there is strikethrough onto a bandage or secondary dressing, the dressing should be changed. Strikethrough provides the ideal vehicle for bacteria to 'travel' along to get to the wound, and it also suggests that the absorptive properties of the primary dressing have been exhausted. Padding over a primary dressing is particularly important in managing heavily exuding wounds. Gamgee (cotton wool inside a gauze cover) is the cheapest option, but can make the legs very hot. Absorbent pads are also helpful although they can be awkward to secure, especially on leg ulcers. The most user-friendly padding for leg ulcers is orthopaedic Velband™, as it can be wound round the leg like a bandage.

Skin care

The skin on the wound margins is often very vulnerable. This is where new cell activity is occurring, and is vital that further skin breakdown is prevented. Wound margins can be successfully protected by applying a small amount of zinc paste to the skin around the wound edge. The zinc paste must be softened before application; mixing in a little white soft paraffin and liquid paraffin is ideal. Minimizing exudate decreases the likelihood of skin maceration and therefore protects the wound margins.

Skin hygiene is key, especially for chronic wounds. The skin must be carefully dried after washing. Particular attention should be paid to between the toes in leg ulcer patients, as cracks here are ideal sites for bacterial infection (leading to possible cellulitis) and fungal infection (leading to possible athlete's foot). Dry skin needs to be moisturized with a cream or ointment (*NB*: creams contain preservatives that can act as sensitizers in people with leg ulcers and should be avoided), and any eczema should be treated with the relevant topical steroid. The dressings themselves can have an impact on the surrounding skin. Hydrocolloids in particular can pull away delicate surrounding tissue, and caution should be taken in using them if the surrounding skin is vulnerable. Under no circumstances should tape be used to stick a dressing onto delicate skin; this is especially important in patients with leg ulcers. Methods of securing dressings are considered below.

Wound bed
Debridement may be required in order to make the wound bed look healthy and red, and once this has been achieved it must be maintained. Foam, alginate or hydrocolloid dressings may be used. Dressings can stay in place longer for wounds that are only exuding slightly than for heavily exuding wounds. Wounds that are almost healed may be covered with a non-adherent dressing. Film dressings may be helpful on a shallow, non-exuding wound, as long as the surrounding skin is in good condition.

Bandaging

Bandaging is important for two reasons; first, it can help secure dressings, and second, in venous disease it promotes the return flow of blood to the heart.

Tape should not be used to stick dressings in place. Instead, various types of bandages should be utilised. The following example illustrates this.

Compression bandaging
The above technique is suitable for patients with either venous or arterial leg ulcers; however the next step, compression bandaging, depends very much on whether the ulcer is arterial or venous.

> **Example**
> You are dressing a leg ulcer, which requires a piece of Lyfoam™ as
> the primary dressing. It slips off at the first possible opportunity, so
> you need to be inventive with your securing strategy. So . . . first you
> get someone else to hold the lyfoam in place, and then you gently
> (with no tension) use a couple of pieces of gauze unfolded to wrap
> around the Lyfoam™. It is now stable. Next you get some tubinette
> and cut a length big enough for a double layer, and put a single layer
> on from the patient s toes to just below his knee. Then you can apply
> your padding; fortunately you have some Velband™, which you wrap
> gently round from toe to knee. You can secure the top of the
> Velband™ with some tape, and you then pull up the second layer of
> the tubinette (asking the patient if he wants his toes in or out).

The principle behind compression bandaging is that it exerts an inward pressure, which helps the venous return. If compression bandaging were to be applied to a patient with arterial disease it would inhibit the arterial flow still further and cause potential damage. Thus compression bandaging must be applied to venous leg ulcers but not to arterial ulcers. Dressings for arterial ulcers may be finally secured with a piece of tubifast.

Compression bandaging is an art in itself and there are now a number of techniques that are used (e.g. four-layer and short-stretch), but the overriding principles are as follows:

1. Ensure that the leg itself is protected with padding (especially if it is skinny). This also gives the leg a normal shape – thinner at the ankle and wider at the calf. If the leg is not protected with padding or flesh, the bandages can dig in (particularly to the shin) and cause traumatic damage (Morison, 1994). If the leg is not an even shape the pressure applied by the bandage will not be even; there needs to be a pressure gradient from the ankle to the knee.
2. Start by securing the bandage round the ball of the foot just below the little toe, and finish just below the knee. A compression bandage applied starting at the ankle will act as a tourniquet, cutting off blood to the foot.
3. As the bandage is wound up the leg, the overlap should be as per the bandage instructions (usually 50 per cent).
4. Apply tension at the same point on each round as the bandage is wound up the leg – i.e. pull at a certain point to create the pressure, which is then maintained as the bandage is wound round.
5. Secure compression bandages with tape rather than pins, as this is safer.

Patient education and support

Patients with chronic wounds are likely to need long-term support. Once again, a leg ulcer is used for illustration purposes.

Having a leg ulcer is a tiring, painful and demoralizing experience. Patients are often subjected to pain, infections, smell, exudate, reduction in mobility and restrictions to their way of life. For many people there are so many false dawns where it seems that things are getting better only to get worse again that they give up interest and hope. As well as providing the ideal physical environment for the ulcer to get better, nurses need to provide the ideal psychological support.

Pain control is important for helping people's own coping strategies. Pain is clearly an individual experience, but monitoring it with a pain assessment tool is useful to gain a picture of when the pain is worse and what helps it. Many patients try to remain stoical and refuse strong pain relief (especially morphine) as they fear addiction; however, morphine is often very helpful and is not addictive if used properly. Dressing changes are often the most painful times, and giving pain relief prior to this is important for patient comfort. The use of entonox during dressing changes is also very helpful.

Once pain is under control, patients feel more able to do other things and focus on other issues that are important to healing their leg ulcers. Venous disease particularly is common in the obese and weight loss is important, although for many this is difficult because of lack of mobility. Walking is helpful, as it stimulates the calf muscle pump (i.e. the contraction of the calf that occurs whilst walking squeezes the blood within the veins and encourages venous return). When patients are not walking they should ideally have their legs elevated, and for elevation to have any real therapeutic effect the legs should be above the level of the heart. Whilst sitting in a chair with legs up on a stool is better than nothing, it is not the most beneficial position. Ideal positions include lying on the bed with the foot of the bed raised, or lying on the sofa with the feet on the arm at one end and the head supported by pillows.

All of these restrictions, on top of the need for frequent dressing changes, can make a patient with leg ulcers very demoralized. To help maintain the morale of patients it is vital to plan small steps that are likely to be successful, rather than saying 'Oohh, we'll have you sorted in no time!'. For example, a first step may be to control the pain, the next step to clean the wound bed, then to improve the skin quality, then to reduce exudate, etc. Patients need to feel involved in what is happening, and choices about dressings and bandaging need to be taken bearing in mind their comfort and preference.

For those with venous disease healing is a real possibility, but it can take years and requires the patient to be diligent about elevation, dressing regimes and weight control. For those with arterial disease the prognosis is less good. Arterial supply can sometimes be improved through the use of surgical techniques, but these are not always successful. Sometimes amputation is an option and, although clearly not a decision to be taken lightly, some patients will choose it rather than continuing to suffer the pain, smell and exudate.

Pressure sores (pressure ulcers)

The pressure sore is the result of impairment of the vascular and lymphatic systems of the skin and deeper tissues caused by the development of compression, tension and shear forces above a critical value and acting for a period of time in tissues between the skeleton and a surface supporting the body.

This definition from Scales (1990) identifies the key elements of pressure sore causation:

1. Impairment of the vascular/lymphatic system
2. Pressure of different types causing this impairment
3. The time over which the pressure is applied has a vital impact.

This is not to exclude other factors, but pressure sores will not form unless the above are present.

In recent years pressure sores have become known, more scientifically, as pressure ulcers. This is appropriate because a sore caused by pressure behaves in the same way as an ulcer caused by vascular insufficiency. Indeed, when considering the healing of an ulcer many of the principles that need to be applied are the same regardless of whether the ulcer is caused by pressure or by vascular deterioration.

It is not the aim here to cover all the elements of pressure ulcer management in huge depth, but the following will be highlighted:

• How do pressure ulcers develop?
• What else contributes to pressure ulcers besides pressure?
• How can pressure ulcers be prevented?

The principles discussed in the previous section on healing ulcers are relevant for management of pressure ulcers.

How do pressure ulcers develop?

Broadly speaking, pressure ulcers develop because of pressure between a bony part of the body, the skin tissues and a surface. Pressure is at its greatest when the bony part of the body is most prominent, the skin tissues are least substantial and the surface is hard.

The first visible sign following pressure on tissues is blanching hyperaemia, which is a reddened area that blanches to pressure. The fact that the skin blanches to pressure shows that no permanent damage has been done, but should indicate that action to protect the pressure areas is needed. The next stage is non-blanching hyperaemia, which is more serious.

Non-blanching hyperaemia is the first sign that pressure exerted on the body has caused damage. This is seen when the skin remains red after pressure has been removed. When pressed with a finger, the redness does not blanch. Although the skin does not show any other outward signs of damage, the fact that the area does not blanch under pressure indicates that underlying tissue damage has already occurred. Urgent action to prevent further breakdown is needed.

Should this urgent action not be forthcoming, the capillaries and lymphatic vessels in the area will burst, causing localized oedema. This is followed by a lack of oxygen in the tissues and a build-up of waste products, which together lead to tissue death. Even at this point the epidermis may remain intact. The underlying tissues will look purplish in colour and feel soft and spongy. It is only a matter of time before the skin breaks down and the purplish area turns to black, necrotic, hard tissue. Thus direct pressure may or may not initially break the epidermis, but any signs of non-blanching hyperaemia must be taken very seriously and immediate preventative action taken if a pressure ulcer is to be prevented.

Shearing forces are also dangerous for patients prone to pressure ulcers. The opposing forces exerted between the patient and the sheets by the patient sliding down the bed can cause tearing of the tissue structures and the microcirculation. A similar situation to that described above can occur, but in addition shearing may cause excoriation and blistering.

What else contributes to pressure ulcers besides pressure?

There are numerous factors that could potentially contribute towards the development of a pressure ulcer. However, the

European Pressure Ulcer Advisory Panel (EPUAP) (1998) gives useful advice and guidance about factors regarding the patient that should be included in any risk assessment. These are:

- General medical condition
- Skin assessment
- Mobility
- Moistness of the skin
- Nutrition
- Pain.

It is worth considering each of these factors in a little more detail.

General medical condition
Key conditions that are particular risk factors are as follows:

- Reduced circulation as, for example, in peripheral vascular disease; this will mean that tissues are less well nourished (i.e. lack of oxygen and nutrients) and therefore more prone to break down.
- Diabetic neuropathy; this leads to reduced sensation, particularly in the extremities, so diabetics may be less aware of damage occurring – particularly to their feet.
- Depression and apathy; this lead to decreased activity and therefore increased susceptibility to pressure.
- Use of certain drugs; some drugs will sedate patients, leading to obvious immobility and the inherent risks this brings. Steroids will thin the skin, making it more delicate and easily broken, and cytotoxics alter the immune system so that fighting infection is less efficient.
- Neurological deficit; for example, a stroke will cause loss of sensation and/or loss of mobility.

Skin assessment
The quality of the skin is vital in determining the susceptibility to pressure ulcers. Dry, brittle or over-wet skin are all more likely to break down. The old ritual of rubbing methylated spirits into heels to harden them did indeed achieve this, but made them more likely to crack. Vigorous rubbing has been a long-held solution for reddened areas on sacrums; however, the EPUAP (1998) is clear that this practice, particularly when carried out on bony prominences, is more likely to cause harm than good as the delicate underlying microcirculation may be disrupted. What is good practice is to ensure that the skin remains in a healthy condition by applying the appropriate moisturizer to clean, dry skin (see Chapter 2). The skin condition must be inspected regularly and

documented clearly within the patients' notes. A good Polaroid photograph is often useful for documenting the skin, although a scale must be placed on the skin.

Mobility

Encouraging mobility is the single most effective way of preventing pressure ulcers. It is useful to examine what pressures are exerted on an individual who is sitting or lying down. There are three factors that need to be taken into account (Phillips, 1997):

1. Vertical pressure, which is 'pressure passing straight down from point of contact to underlying bone and compressing all tissue in between'. Therefore the greatest pressure is likely to occur over bony areas.
2. Interface pressure, which is a pressure exerted in the opposite direction from the vertical pressure, representing the force applied by whatever it is being sat or laid upon. Interface pressure is related to the patient's weight and can be expressed by the equation:

Interface pressure = weight/surface area supported

   Interface pressure can be visualized by imagining an overweight woman in stiletto heels. Her mass is large and the surface area for support small, thus leading to a large interface pressure on the feet (and the floor). To minimize interface pressure, the general principle must be to spread the weight over a large surface area. This is what roho cushions achieve.
3. Capillary closing pressure is the pressure at which the capillaries shut down, thus preventing blood from circulating to the tissues. Historically this pressure has been fixed at 32 mmHg (Landis, 1930), but it is now thought that other factors (such as how ill the patient is) may lower this further. As this pressure is physiologically fixed there is not a lot that the nurse can do to change it; however, by reducing the other two pressures the likelihood of reaching the capillary closing pressure will be reduced.

Moistness of the skin

There will be little doubt in most nurses' minds that incontinent patients are at greater risk of skin breakdown and pressure ulcers than those who are continent. It is thought that it is not that ammonia in urine that acts as a major component in skin breakdown, but rather the moisture. Faecal incontinence, on the other hand, is thought to act as an irritant (Kemp, 1994). Excessive moisture in combination with friction from bedding act to make the skin more vulnerable. Thus, preventative strategies of careful washing and, most importantly, drying are vital to protect the skin.

Le Lievre (1996), in a review of the evidence on managing incontinence, advocates the use of super-absorbent pads that will draw the moisture away from the skin. She recommends that washing is not necessary following urinary incontinence if super-absorbent pads are being used, and washing with water only is required if normal pads are used. As discussed in Chapter 2 over-washing with soap can alter the skin's normal ability to maintain integrity.

It is worth remembering that very sweaty (e.g. pyrexial) patients are at similar risk. A further point is that hot, wet skin is an ideal environment for fungal and bacterial infections, which can themselves cause the skin to crack and become sore.

Nutrition

A thin patient with more exaggerated bony prominences will be subject to greater vertical pressures and thus more prone to pressure ulcers. However, an obese person will be subject to greater interface pressures and more likely to have delayed mobility following surgery/trauma, thus increasing their risk of pressure ulcers. Being at either end of the weight spectrum puts an individual at risk. The condition of the skin is affected by how well hydrated the body is, and therefore adequate fluid intake is important. The impact of other nutritional elements on the development of pressure ulcers is contentious, although clearly a balanced diet is needed to maintain general well-being.

Pain

Pain is likely to be a risk factor when it causes reduced mobility. This is for two reasons: first, it may prevent someone from getting out of bed and moving because doing so is too painful; and second, at a microlevel extreme pain may decrease the number of small movements someone makes whilst sitting or lying still. Itch is often not considered in assessment tools; however, itch can mean that an individual will scratch so much that the skin surface is damaged and therefore the likelihood of developing a pressure ulcer is increased.

Nursing care

The most fundamentally important part of pressure ulcer care is prevention. This must be done through an understanding of pressure ulcer formation and the risk factors involved. Nursing action must take place as part of the multidisciplinary team;

physiotherapists and occupational therapists in particular will have much to contribute to pressure ulcer prevention. Patients should be encouraged to do as much for themselves as possible, and wherever possible carers should be taught to be vigilant for skin deterioration.

As far as possible, practice must be evidence-based. In the case of pressure ulcers this may not always be possible. A Royal College of Nursing document on pressure ulcer assessment and prevention highlights the fact that much practice is based on limited scientific evidence (RCN, 2001). This document provides invaluable guidance on which parts of the practice related to this area are based on acceptable scientific study and which are gained from expert consensus. The following list highlights key elements of nursing care in this area.

1. *Reduce pressure to a minimum.* The best way of doing this is to encourage patients to move, preferably by mobilizing, but if this is impossible, by making small shifts of weight in the bed or chair. Nursing time tends to be dedicated to turning patients whilst they are in bed, but helping patients to stand once they are sitting in a chair often receives less attention. Pressure exerted on vulnerable areas whilst sitting in a chair can be high, especially if the chair fits the patient badly. Planting the feet firmly on the floor or on a footrest relieves some of the pressure from the ischial tuberosities, whereas having the legs dangling means that all the pressure is going through the back of the legs and the buttocks. If a patient's feet are up on a stool, it is important to be vigilant about the pressure exerted on the heels; their bony nature means that they are extremely vulnerable.
2. *Keep the skin clean, dry and supple* – follow the advice given in this book!
3. *Make an initial assessment of the skin and continually update it.* There is a range of assessment tools available, but it is important that the one chosen covers all the elements laid down by the EPUAP. The Medley Score (Williams, 1991) fulfils all the criteria and is very specific in many areas (e.g. nutrition, continence and skin), but it is less specific in the general medical area. Waterlow (1987) provides more detail regarding medical conditions. Choice of which score is suitable is dependent on the clinical area; however, assessments should not be limited to 'on admission' but be performed as part of an ongoing process. Flanagan (1997) highlights seven potential problems with the pressure ulcer at-risk assessment tools, and if clinical areas can acknowledge and where possible tackle these

problems, the use of such tools is likely to be more effective:

- Validity and reliability of the tool is often not proven
- The tool may be inappropriate for the clinical setting
- Staff may be unfamiliar with it
- There may be inconsistent re-evaluation of the patient's risk status
- There may be inconsistent documentation of the risk status and preventative care in the nursing notes
- There may be failure to implement appropriate preventive/ treatment plans once the risk status has been identified
- There may be an over-reliance on identified risk status combined with the failure of nursing staff to use their own judgement.

Observation of the skin during the assessment period may indicate that damage has already occurred. Grading systems for pressure ulcers can be a useful way of monitoring skin breakdown, although they differ in their approaches to the stages of skin deterioration, which can be confusing. Torrance (1983) includes blanching hyperaemia (Table 3.2), whereas the Surrey grading system (David *et al.*, 1983; Table 3.3) does not. The decision regarding which system to use will need to be made with the types of patients being cared for in mind.
4. *Give due regard to the medical condition* – see above.

When considering pressure ulcers, prevention should be the main aim of care. Should an ulcer develop, the sooner it is identified and action taken the more likely it is that treatment will be successful. Application of good skin care will help to reduce the likelihood of skin deterioration and therefore pressure ulcer formation. Nurses must work as part of a multidisciplinary team, using the best evidence available to maximize the impact of care.

Table 3.2 The Torrance grading system for pressure ulcers

Grade	Description
Stage 1	Blanching hyperaemia
Stage 2	Non-blanching hyperaemia
Stage 3	Ulceration progresses through the dermis only
Stage 4	Lesion extends into the subcutaneous fat
Stage 5	Infective necrosis penetrates the deep fascia

Table 3.3 The Surrey grading system for pressure ulcers

Grade	Description
Stage 1	Non-blanching hyperaemia
Stage 2	Superficial break in the skin
Stage 3	Destruction of skin without cavity
Stage 4	Destruction of the skin with cavity

Contact dermatitis

Contact dermatitis describes the reaction of the skin to an external substance that acts as an allergen or an irritant. Contact dermatitis is an occupational hazard, as many of the substances that people come into contact with in their working lives can cause an undesirable reaction. Occupational contact dermatitis is thought to account for up to 37 per cent of the occupational illnesses in the USA (Stewart *et al.*, 1992).

Contact dermatitis is a particularly important consideration in people with skin disease. Skin disease means that there are more likely to be breaks in the skin, and an individual is at higher risk of developing an allergic contact sensitization as the allergen can easily penetrate the skin's protective layer. Also, atopic individuals (i.e. those with underlying atopic eczema) are 13.5 times more likely to develop contact dermatitis than those without atopic eczema (Shmunes and Keil, 1984).

Clear distinction needs to be made between the different mechanisms that cause contact dermatitis.

Allergic reactions

Allergic reactions involve an immunological response to contact with an external substance. A Type I reaction is immediate; histamine is released, causing hives, rhinoconjunctivitis (streaming eyes) and, more seriously, angioedema and anaphylaxis. The reaction can last for up to 2 hours, and can clearly be life threatening. A Type IV reaction, which is more common, involves the body becoming sensitized to a substance (antigen) over a period of time. The substance penetrates the skin barrier, where the Langerhans cells attach to the antigen and 'present' it to the T lymphocyte helper cells. These are then expanded in the lymph node so that T-effector and T-memory cells are released into the bloodstream. This process of sensitization can take between 5 and 21 days. Following this first exposure there is no outward reaction, but on subsequent exposure the sensitized T cells migrate to the point of contact, causing inflammation. This normally takes 48–72 hours. An allergic reaction may cause an overall rash rather than one just at the point of contact (Plotnick, 1990).

Irritant reactions

An irritant reaction is a non-immunological reaction that occurs when a substance comes into contact with the skin. An acute reaction occurs immediately following contact with substances such as acids and alkalis, whereas more cumulative effects occur following prolonged contact with such things as soaps and solvents.

It can be difficult to distinguish between allergic and irritant dermatitis, and indeed difficult to ascertain exactly what is causing the dermatitis. Patch testing is a way of determining what is causing contact dermatitis, although this usually needs to be done within a dermatology department. It involves taking an in-depth history to gain a picture of the sorts of things someone may be reacting to. Then a number of chemicals commonly found in everyday substances, alongside substances related to an individual's occupation, are placed in small metal chambers and stuck onto the back (Plates 1 and 2). The concentrations and quantities are such that irritant reactions should be kept to a minimum, but these can still occur. Readings are taken at 48 hours and then at 72+ hours, the time lapse allowing the allergic reaction to occur (Swartz and Sherertz, 1993). This is why, when trying out a new cream or ointment on a patient, a small patch test should be performed and left for 48 hours to be sure that an allergic reaction is not going to take place.

Patients with chronic leg ulcers are particularly at risk of developing allergic reactions. When the skin barrier function is breached, there is a particular risk of absorbing allergens from dressings and topical applications (Cameron *et al.*, 1992). A study by Wilson *et al.* (1991) showed that 23 per cent of leg ulcer patients were allergic to wool alcohols found in lanolin, but more recent work has shown that modern techniques have allowed lanolin to be 'purified' to the extent where it has virtually no allergenic properties (Wright, 1999). However, there is still concern about the use of cream emollients for patients with leg ulcers, as their preservatives can act as allergens. Using ointment-based emollients for patients with leg ulcers is always safest.

Although patch testing is a very useful way of identifying substances that might be causing contact dermatitis it is not infallible, as placing small amounts of chemical on the back of individuals does not recreate the environment they find themselves in at work. However, if positives are found then advice must be given about avoiding this substance. This can be particularly difficult if the substance is a very common one like latex.

Latex allergy

Latex allergy is becoming more common, and is a real problem for many nurses. For some the allergy is caused by the leaching out of chemicals that are used during the manufacture of the gloves. This is likely to lead to Type IV reactions. A Type I allergy is likely to occur in someone who has an allergy to latex itself, and for these people the only solution is to wear latex-free gloves. It is worth noting that some brands of glove claim to be hypoallergenic, which means they contain lower amounts of the chemicals from manufacture, but they are not latex free (Townsend, 1994). Some patients are allergic to latex and will react when touched by a latex glove, and normally these people will carry a warning card. However, it is becoming more common practice for health care workers to avoid latex gloves altogether.

Protection

When it is impossible for an individual to avoid the substance that causes the contact dermatitis (e.g. a car mechanic who is sensitized to oil), other strategies must be employed. These involve wearing protective gloves, careful washing of hands, and wearing barrier creams or ointments. It can be very distressing for patients to find that it is their job that is causing the skin problem, especially if an acute allergy means that the only option is to give up the job. However, it can also be a major relief to find the cause of what in some cases amounts to years of suffering. For most people, discussion with the occupational health department in their workplace and careful skin care can lead to a solution that allows the individual to carry on working.

Skin changes due to dermatological conditions

There are over a thousand different dermatological conditions, but the most common by far are skin cancers, acne, eczema, psoriasis and infective lesions. Skin cancers and acne have already been considered in this book (see above and Chapter 2), so this chapter concentrates on the other broad categories, as these are most likely to be seen in a general setting. Although diseases are described, nursing deficits in self-care are highlighted along with the appropriate nursing actions.

Psoriasis

Psoriasis affects approximately 2 per cent of the population, and does not appear to have any gender bias. It is unusual (although not impossible) for it to present in childhood or adolescence; the first signs are generally seen in the second or third decade of life.

Presentation

Psoriasis usually presents as red, scaly plaques that describe a slightly raised area of skin with a well-defined edge. Whilst the plaques themselves are pinkish-red, they are covered with a layer of silvery skin scales (Plate 3). In dark skin the plaques will appear darker in colour and not so distinctly pinkish-red, but they will still have the distinctive layer of silver skin scales. In theory psoriasis can affect any part of the body, but in practice it rarely occurs on the face. It is often symmetrical, so if there is a plaque on one knee there is likely to be one on the other.

Psoriasis can also occur under the nails. If this happens the psoriasis pushes the nail up from the nail bed, causing it to separate and lift up, and this is called onycholysis. Psoriasis can also affect the nail as it grows, causing pitting, which appears as little indentations in the nails (du Vivier, 1997). Some patients also suffer from psoriatic arthritis, which causes painful joints, particularly in the distal interphalangeal joints of the fingers and small joints of the toes (Baker, 1989).

Although psoriasis normally presents as plaques (small or large) it can, in very serious cases, become erythrodermic, where the whole body is covered by hot, extremely scaly skin (Plate 4). This is unusual but can be life threatening, especially for those with cardiac failure. The metabolic activity required to keep erythrodermic skin active is huge, and can therefore put a dangerous stress on the cardiac system.

Causes

The exact cause of psoriasis has not been unequivocally established. It is believed that there is an immunological fault which causes the skin to develop at a rate 10 times that of normal skin. The daughter cells produced by the basal layer of the epidermis progress to the stratum corneum in 2–3 days rather than the normal 30 and build up into the plaques which are visible to eye. Psoriatic skin cells do not go through the final stages of maturation and do not produce the Odland bodies which make the natural oil that helps to hold the stratum corneum together. This explains why the plaques are covered in dry scale that sheds constantly and visibly.

For a lot of people psoriasis has long periods of remission where there are no visible lesions. There is thought to be a definite genetic component to the disease and whilst for some, psoriasis may run in the family this is by no means always the case. The reasons why psoriasis suddenly develops are not properly understood either, however some "trigger factors" have been identified. Sometimes psoriasis is triggered by certain drugs e.g. lithium and chloroquine. Physical trauma may cause psoriasis to develop for example along the line of a surgical incision, this is known as Koebners phenomenon. Many people report that stress triggers their psoriasis but this is not always so. Upper respiratory tract infection is known to trigger a particular type of psoriasis known as guttate psoriasis which is distinct because of a widespread distribution of small papular plaques.

Symptoms

Symptoms will of course vary from person to person, but there are some common symptoms that many people report:

1. Irritation – the plaques often feel itchy and the temptation is to scratch, although this will cause bleeding
2. Soreness – this may be because individuals have scratched the plaques so much, or because the skin has become so dry that it cracks
3. Stress – the psoriasis itself often causes individuals to feel stressed as they have to cope with treating it and the reactions of others around them, which often causes embarrassment (Penzer, 1994)
4. Scaliness – psoriasis is scaly and means the patient constantly has to cope with falling flakes of skin.

CASE STUDY

Peter Chalmers, a 75-year-old man, is admitted with worsening cardiac failure. He has chronic plaque psoriasis, which he has had since the age of 50. He is short of breath and is finding it very hard to do things for himself. He finds treatment for his psoriasis particularly hard as it means he has to bend, twist and rub ointments onto parts of his body that are difficult to reach. He is knowledgeable about his skin, but is very worried that now that he is in hospital his skin won t be looked after, as his wife has been helping him at home. He has brought with him a list of the things he uses, which he asks to have written up by the doctor so that the right treatments are available whilst he is in hospital.

Following assessment, the following are identified as areas in which Peter has a self-care deficit:

1. *Bathing.* Although Peter can wash himself once he is in the bath, he needs help to prepare the bath and to get into it. There needs to be a measure of bath oil (e.g. Balneum™) put into the bath water, and Peter needs to be able to reach the aqueous cream that he uses to wash himself with. When he washes his hair Peter uses a special shampoo, called Polytar™, which helps to control the psoriasis in his scalp. He needs help drying himself, which should be done by patting or very gently rubbing dry.

2. *Moisturing.* Immediately after the bath Peter likes to have his moisturizer applied. He uses a light moisturizing cream called Cetraben™, as his psoriasis is not too bad at the moment. He can apply this to his arms and front, but needs help to apply it to his back. Peter explains to the nurse that although he only needs to apply the cream to his plaques he likes to apply it all over, as he finds that it keeps the rest of his skin in good condition and slows down the development of new plaques. Peter shows the nurse how to apply the cream in a downward motion following the line of the hair.

3. *Treatment.* Peter is using a cream called Alphosyl™. This is a weak tar-based preparation that is applied twice daily to the plaques. It has to be rubbed in quite carefully, and Peter explains that it is important for the nurse to wear gloves whilst doing this as the Alphosyl™ can be irritating on non-psoriatic skin. He has some psoriasis in his groin, which Peter treats himself. He does not use the tar preparation here due to the delicate nature of the skin, and instead uses a weak topical steroid ointment. Peter does have some psoriasis in his scalp, which needs massaging with coconut oil. This is best done at night before going to bed as he does not like wandering round during the day with greasy hair. Applying the coconut oil involves parting the hair into sections and rubbing the ointment in along the parting (see Chapter 2).

4. *Dressing.* Peter can get dressed independently, although it takes him a long time. When he is using Alphosyl™, which is a bit smelly and quite greasy, he always wears old clothes, but to stop the ointment coming off he uses tubifast on his limbs and an old cotton vest for his trunk.

5. *Comfort.* During the day Peter can manage not to scratch his skin even though it does irritate. However, at night he finds it much harder not to scratch and has been taking a drug with an antipruritic effect (hydroxyzine).

6. *Coping.* Peter has got used to his psoriasis and does not let it bother him in day-to-day life. The help that he requires in hospital is that the staff listen to what he needs and help him to maintain his regime as normally as possible.

General principles of treatment

Although there are a variety of other treatments for psoriasis, the general principles remain the same as outlined in the above case study. Moisturizing at least once and usually twice a day is a must, followed by careful application of the active topical medication. It is important to remember that the topical preparations, including the moisturizers, are drugs and need to be prescribed in the same way as any other drug. There are a number of topical applications suitable for the treatment of psoriasis; however, they generally belong to one of the following categories:

1. Tar. This can come in a relatively purified form, which decreases the smell. However, there is always a slight smell associated with it and a tendency to mark clothing when it is first applied. Some examples included Alphosyl™, Exorex™ lotion and Cocois™ (scalp application).
2. Dithranol. This is a synthetically prepared product, the origins of which are found in tree bark. It is effective for well-defined psoriasis, as great care is needed on application because it irritates normal skin. Careful instructions need to be followed, as some types of dithranol need to be washed off 30 minutes after application. Examples include Dithrocream™ and Micanol™.
3. Vitamin D analogues. These creams and ointments are odourless and easy to apply. They affect the way that cells develop and stop the process of overproduction. They can cause transient irritation on application. Examples include Dovonex™ and Curatoderm™.
4. Vitamin A analogues. These are relatively new, and once again suppress cell activity. Irritation on application is a possible problem. An example is Zorac™.
5. Topical steroids. These are not, on the whole, the treatment of choice for psoriasis. They tend to suppress rather than stop the increased cell proliferation, which means that, particularly when potent steroids are used, once they are withdrawn the psoriasis often returns. However, topical steroids are very useful for treating inflamed psoriasis and areas that are too delicate for other topical applications.

Although Peter is not taking systemic therapy in the case study above, in severe cases of psoriasis this is necessary. Some examples of systemic drugs include: methotrexate, a cytotoxic which limits the cell proliferation; retinoid, a vitamin A analogue that affects skin cell synthesis; and cyclosporin, an immunosuppressive that stops the skin cells from proliferating (Gilleaudeau and McClelland, 1994).

Atopic eczema

(Note that this is different from contact eczema, which is discussed earlier in this chapter, and that dermatitis can be used interchangeably with the word eczema.)

Atopic eczema is most prevalent in children, with 14 per cent of those under 12 years of age suffering from it (Bysshe, 1996). Although some adults continue to suffer with atopic eczema, 90 per cent of affected children have outgrown it by their mid-teens (Bysshe, 1996). Children who suffer from asthma and hay fever seem to be more prone to eczema.

Presentation

Atopic eczema presents in a number of different ways. Chronic eczema presents as dry, scaling skin, often with exaggerated skin markings known as lichenification. Acute eczema is inflamed, red, often weeping, and sometimes has vesicles or blisters (Perkins, 1996). In infancy eczema often appears initially on the face, but other common locations in later childhood are the flexures of the elbows and the knees, and on the wrists and ankles (Donald, 1995). In adults eczema is often seen on the hands. In the older patient venous stasis causes eczema on the lower legs, often accompanied by ulceration.

Causes

Eczema is a genetically inherited disease that, like psoriasis, has a series of trigger factors that make it more active. Trigger factors depend on the individual, and some people will be more sensitive than others, but common factors include house dust mite and infection. *Staphylococcus aureus* is particularly common in eczematous lesions, and is often responsible for eczema worsening (Perkins, 1996).

Symptoms

The degree to which people suffer with the following will vary, but most people with atopic eczema will report:

1. Irritation. This is a major problem for everyone with eczema. Scratching is a common response and is often subconscious, and the results of scratching include:

   - Worsening itch (itch–scratch cycle)
   - Smooth/shiny nails from rubbing and scratching
   - Shortened, stubby body hairs that have broken due to constant scratching
   - Infection as the scratching causes breaks in the skin.

2. Soreness. As a result of the above the skin becomes sore; some people would rather have sore than itchy skin, and therefore scratch until their skin becomes painful. Acute eczema is often sore without having been scratched.

3. Stress. The appearance of eczema can be very embarrassing, particularly if it is weeping. It is not uncommon for eczema to be so irritating that it disrupts sleep patterns. In families where children have eczema it can put enormous strain on family relationships as members struggle to cope with treatments and sleepless nights (Lawson *et al.*, 1999).

CASE STUDY

Emma Stubbs is a 22-year-old woman who has come in for stabilization of her asthma following a serious exacerbation of her condition. Although she has had atopic eczema since childhood she has not been troubled by it in the last 5 years. On talking to her, the admitting nurse realizes that she has very little awareness about her treatments. She has a big bag of tubes and tubs, but only the vaguest idea about how to use them. She is very depressed about the state of her skin, particularly as she has just started a new relationship and is acutely aware of how she looks. Initially she seems not to care about doing treatments herself, and it becomes clear that the nurse s job is going to be one of education and support.

Having decided that education is a key part of Emma s care, the nurse decides to wait until Emma is able to breathe more normally before focusing on teaching her about caring for her skin. As Emma becomes more comfortable with her breathing it is possible to plan her skin care with her. Although Emma is now capable of self-caring, most of her deficits lie in the fact that her knowledge is confused and limited. The nurse decides to find out what is normal for Emma and help her to develop a treatment regime around this, and the following advice is given:

1. *Bathing*. Emma usually showers in the evening before going to bed, so advising her to continue doing this but to use an emollient shower gel, such as Oilatum™ shower gel, allows her to stick to her routine. She is very keen to rub herself vigorously afterwards to stop the itching, so an explanation about how this might actually damage the skin and make it itchier is important.

2. *Moisturizing*. Emma hates the feel of very greasy ointments on her skin, but she is willing to try anything new. In this situation Epaderm™ is a good choice, as although it is very greasy it sinks in well. Emma will need to apply it liberally in a downward motion all over her body. Because it is relatively greasy it is best to use it at night before going to bed, and then to wear old

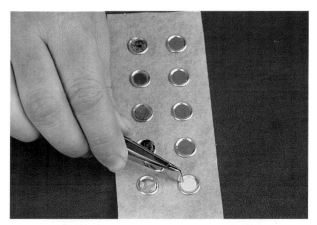

Plate 1. Patch test chambers being prepared

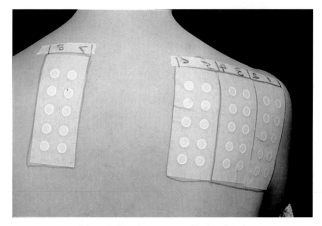

Plate 2. Patch tests applied to back

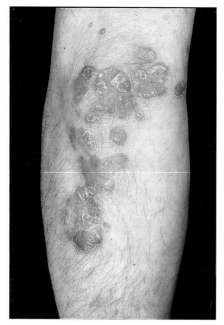

Plate 3. Plaque psoriasis on knee

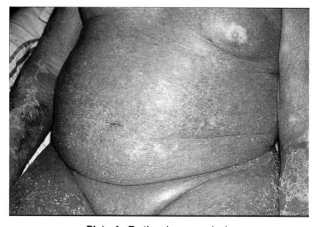

Plate 4. Erythroderm psoriasis

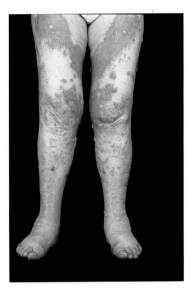

Plate 5. Bullous pemphigoid

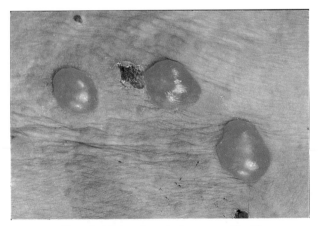

Plate 6. Blisters from bullous pemphigoid

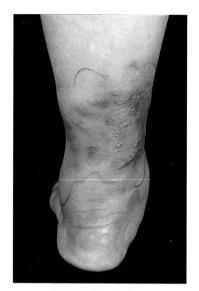

Plate 7. Erysipelas

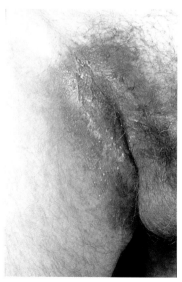

Plate 8. Candidiasis fungal
infection in groin

nightclothes and/or cover her limbs with tubifast. The latter has the advantage, as it makes it harder to scratch the skin. A lighter moisturizer, e.g. Cetraben™, might be used during the day. She should take this to work with her and apply it as often as she can. Emma is worried about her boyfriend s reactions to her going to bed with greasy skin. It is important to reassure her that although the greasy emollients are best, the important thing is that she applies some moisturizer. If it is not always the greasy one, this is not a major problem.

3. *Steroids*. Emma is frightened about using topical steroids, as she has heard that they can thin your skin and cause stretch marks. Clear guidance and support about the basic rules of topical steroid use should help to allay these fears (see Chapter 5). It is best if they can be written down:

   • It is much more important (and effective) to use the right amount of strong steroid for a short period of time rather than smaller, weaker amounts over a longer period
   • The right amount can be measured out using fingertip measurements to ensure that the right amount is being used
   • Once the skin gets better it is advisable to use a weaker potency of steroid and then gradually wean off it by using it less frequently
   • Always use a moisturizer before using steroids as this will reduce the amount that is needed and enable it to sink in more effectively
   • Use less potent steroids on delicate parts of the skin (e.g. the face and skin folds).

4. *Occlusion*. Although Emma tries hard not to, she cannot help scratching. She does keep her nails short and takes antipruritics before going to bed, although she complains they make her drowsy the following morning. Using occlusion (i.e. wrapping the affected areas to stop her from scratching and to enhance the action of the topical therapies) is a useful possible solution. Occlusion can be something simple such as tubifast on limbs, or can be more complex paste bandaging. This involves applying bandages impregnated with medicaments (e.g. coal tar, zinc paste or icthamol) next to the skin. The bandages need to be applied carefully and not just wound round the limb; instead they need to be pleated in a backwards and forwards motion. It is important to apply them in this way because when they dry they contract, and if they are just wound around the limb they will act as a tourniquet. They act to soothe the skin, and make it very difficult to scratch.

5. *At home*. Once Emma gets home it is advisable for her to continue with the regime as taught to her. Once the acute attack has subsided she can stop using the steroids, but she will need

> to continue to use the moisturizers. You advise her to try and keep house dust to a minimum by regular vacuuming and damp dusting, and by minimizing the number of soft furnishings in the house. She should try to keep cool and should wear cotton garments wherever possible. Avoiding very perfumed things such as cosmetics or fabric softeners is also advisable.

General principles of treatment

The treatment outlined for Emma above is the standard treatment for eczema. Emollients and steroids remain the mainstays. Education and support are also important, as it can be very confusing trying to understand which of the many topical applications have to be applied to the various different parts of the skin. As with psoriasis, in serious cases systemic drugs may be used – most commonly cyclosporin, an immunosuppressant. It is not uncommon for patients with eczema to be on oral antibiotics; these can often have a dramatic effect on clearing up the skin, thus indicating the significant role that bacterial infection has in exacerbating eczema.

Blisters

Blisters are an accumulation of fluid lying within the epidermis or immediately under it. There are many causes of skin blistering, including some viral infections, such as herpes zoster (shingles); acute dermatitis; and allergies to some plants, such as poison ivy or primula. Blistering is particularly common in the most acute phase of the disease. For example, although eczema often looks dry and scaly, in an acute flare-up the skin can blister and small vesicles form. However, there are a number of specific diseases where blisters are the main symptom (e.g. pemphigus vulgaris and dermatitis herpatiformis) and these diseases are autoimmune in nature. There are a number of blistering conditions, which all present in slightly different ways and affect different sections of the population. The most common blistering condition, bullous pemphigoid, is examined in more detail here. This mainly affects those over the age of 60 years, and there do not seem to be any other predisposing factors.

Presentation

Pemphigoid presents as firm, tense blisters, which can appear all over the body but do not tend to affect the mucous membranes (Plate 5). Before the blisters appear an individual may describe erythematous, itchy, slightly raised areas that have no other obvious cause (Graham-Brown and Burns, 1990) (Plate 6). Once pemphigoid has appeared it can be difficult to get under control, and a patient may get new blisters for weeks or even months. However, control can be achieved with the correct drug therapy and a patient can experience periods of remission when they have no symptoms, although it can recur.

Causes
Nobody is sure of the exact cause of blistering disorders, but what is certain is that there are some immunological changes that cause the layers of the skin to split away from one another. In pemphigoid, this split happens at the junction between the epidermis and dermis. (By way of comparison, a friction blister involves the skin splitting in the layers of the epidermis.)

Symptoms
Pemphigoid is initially itchy and can become sore once the blisters are open, especially if they are in areas that tend to experience pressure (e.g. the sacrum). The condition can be extremely unsightly, and very worrying for the patient.

CASE STUDY

Mary Peters, a 64-year-old woman, is admitted to the ward with bullous pemphigoid. She was diagnosed with this condition a year ago. It had been under control, but in the last week new blisters have been appearing and Mary and her district nurse have not been able to cope with them. Mary is a very knowledgeable person and is well aware of the implications of the new blisters. She is drinking plenty of fluids to counterbalance fluid loss, and keeping the blisters clean to minimize the likelihood of infection. She has been told that she will have to increase the amount of oral steroid she is taking from 10 mg daily to 80 mg a day, which she is unhappy about, but she understands the need to suppress her immune system to stop new blisters forming. The admitting nurse discusses the situation with Mary, and they decide that her self-care deficits are in the following areas:

1. *Safety.* Due to the high level of steroids that Mary is on, she is at risk of steroid-induced hypertension and diabetes. It is important to measure Mary s blood pressure once a week and also to test her urine for sugar once a week. As already mentioned, Mary is at risk of secondary infection because of the open blisters, and this is made more likely by the fact that she is being immunosuppressed by the drugs. Mary knows what her

skin looks like when the blisters are infected, and is capable of helping to monitor for signs of infection.

2. *Hygiene*. Although Mary can get in and out of the bath by herself, she needs some help in preparing it. This involves providing aqueous cream for washing and dissolving potassium permanganate in the bath. This is mildly antiseptic and also helps to dry the exuding blisters. (The potassium permanganate crystals must be carefully dissolved in very hot water first to ensure that they dissolve properly. Only a tiny amount on the end of a spatula should be used enough to turn the bath water light pink. It is preferable to use the tablets, which are ready measured and dissolve more safely.)

3. *Steroids*. As well as taking steroids orally, Mary needs to have topical steroids applied to her skin. Before applying the steroids the blisters need to be burst and drained, counting the number of new blisters each day to monitor the activity of the disease. (Once the number of new blisters begins to decrease the disease is being treated effectively.) A scalpel should be used to slit the underside of the blisters and the exudate absorbed with gauze. A potent form of topical steroid is then applied to the lesions. New wet lesions respond most effectively to the cream formulation of the steroid, whereas the older blister sites are best treated with the ointment formulation, and the presentation of the steroid will alter depending on the state of the blister. Mary can demonstrate the sorts of non-adherent dressings that she and the district nurse use to cover the blisters. She explains that the best way to hold them in place is with tubifast; using tape on her skin can damage it further, and wrapping cotton conforming bandages around a limb can act as a tourniquet.

4. *Support*. Mary and her family will need a positive and knowledgeable approach. They are very worried that they may have to cope with flare-ups every year, and it is impossible to guarantee that they will not. However, reassurance needs to be given that longer periods of remission are possible. Indeed it is possible that the disease may be self-limiting so that no further treatment is necessary, but it can take up to 5 years for this to happen (Graham-Brown and Burns, 1990).

General principles of treatment

The treatments for bullous pemphigoid centre on immunosuppression. Topical and oral steroids are always used, and often other immunosuppressants such as azathioprine are added to the regime. Maintaining patient safety in terms of monitoring for infection and the side effects of drugs is crucial, as is giving lots of psychological support.

Infections

The human skin is covered in commensal bacteria and fungi that are vital for preventing pathogenic organisms from causing disease. Indeed, of the millions (10^{14}) of cells that make up our being, only 10 per cent are human and the rest are commensal organisms (Savin, 1998). Cutaneous infections happen when the balance of commensal organisms is disrupted, or when a breach in the skin integrity allows an organism to penetrate the skin's protective surface.

Cutaneous infections can be broadly divided into three groups; bacterial, fungal and viral.

Bacterial infections

There are a number of different bacterial infections of the skin, but the two most common groups are those caused by staphylococcal and streptococcal bacteria.

Generally all bacterial infections are more likely to occur where standards of hygiene are low and when the climate is hot and wet. *S. aureus* is responsible for causing impetigo, ecthyma and folliculitis. Impetigo is usually seen in children, and ecthyma in those who are immunodepressed. It is sometimes a progression from impetigo or folliculitis. Folliculitis is often caused by treatments for dry skin (see Chapter 2).

Any one can develop a streptococcal skin infection, although the elderly, and particularly those with leg ulceration, are particularly at risk.

Presentation
Impetigo presents as vesicles which, when scratched, rupture and produce a honey-coloured crust. It normally occurs on exposed surfaces, in particular on the face.

Ecthyma presents as multiple shallow round ulcers, which sometimes progress into deeper ulcers.

Folliculitis presents as pustules that develop around the hair follicles, and often have a hair protruding out of the centre of them.

Erysipelas, which describes a dermal streptococcal infection, presents as well-defined erythematous and often swollen areas (Plate 7). There may be some associated lymphadenopathy when erysipelas affects a limb, and if it occurs on the face oedema around the eyes is not unusual. The oedema may be complicated by blood blisters.

Cellulitis describes a streptococcal infection that has gone deeper, causing darker red lesions and more significant oedema.

Causes

Impetigo is often seen on children with itchy skin (either because of scabies or eczema) who scratch it with dirty fingernails. It is also associated with discharging middle ear infections.

Ecthyma may develop in those who have a depressed immune system.

Folliculitis occurs when skin follicles are irritated by occlusive greasy treatments.

Streptococcal infections enter the skin via very small breaches of skin integrity, such as in athlete's foot, an insect bite or a small fissure at the corner of the mouth or behind the ears.

Symptoms

In all of the staphylococcal infections there may be some minimal irritation, but the only one that may be painful is ecthyma. Erysipelas and cellulitis are both accompanied by 'flu-like' symptoms and fever. The affected area is likely to be painful and very tender to the touch.

Treatment

Bacterial infections will need treating with antibiotics and good hygiene. A superficial bacterial infection might respond satisfactorily to topical antibiotics, but more usually oral antibiotics will be needed. Topical antibiotics should be used with caution, as they are capable of causing skin sensitivities. It is vital that patients are given information about why they have got an infection and how they can avoid it in the future. This may involve more careful hygiene and/or stopping scratching.

Fungal infections

There are numerous fungal infections that can affect humans. Cutaneous fungal infections include:

- Tinea, which is caused by multicellular fungi that live in the stratum corneum of the skin, hair and nails
- Candidiasis, which is caused by are single cell yeasts that normally live in the mucosae of the gastrointestinal and genital tracts.

Affected populations

Tinea is otherwise known as ringworm, and affects the body or scalp. It is often passed on from animals, and is spread easily among children in schools.

Candidiasis is the general term for infections such as thrush or intertrigo (fungal infections affecting the skin folds) (Plate 8). People who are prone to yeast infections include pregnant women and those on the oral contraceptive pill, people who are immuno-suppressed, those on broad-spectrum antibiotics, diabetics, and people with HIV infection. It is most likely to occur in warm, moist areas of the body.

Presentation

Tinea usually present as a slightly scaly ovoid lesion; if occurring on the scalp, the affected area will be hairless.

Candidiasis will look different depending on where it presents. In the mouth there will be whitish patches, which if scraped away will reveal an inflamed mucosal surface. In the vagina the appearance on the vaginal wall may be similar to the patches in the mouth, although a discharge is more usually the first symptom. In the skin folds (intertrigo), the eruption is moist and erythematous with a well-defined edge; it may be scaly or pustular. Candida can get under the nail and infect the nail bed if the cuticle is damaged. Fungal infection under the nail causes it to become ridged and misshapen.

Causes

Tinea is passed on by coming into contact with keratin debris carrying the fungus. It may be passed from a human to human, or from an animal to human.

Candidiasis is caused by yeasts that exist normally in the body but become a problem (pathogenic) when there is some imbalance in normal body function.

Symptoms

Tinea may be itchy, although this varies. The scaling may be significant. In some people, scalp ringworm may leave permanent bald patches.

Candidiasis in the vagina is always accompanied by itch; elsewhere it may be uncomfortable, especially if the skin cracks, but it is unlikely to be painful.

Treatment

A superficial infection of either tinea or candidiasis will respond to topical antifungal preparations. It is vital that topical preparations are applied diligently and for the correct length of time. If they are stopped when the symptoms start to fade there will be re-infection, as the fungal spores will still be active. Application of topical antifungals must be accompanied by good skin care with special attention to skin folds, which must be washed and, most importantly, dried effectively. Candida infection under the nail is difficult to treat, although oral Lamisil™ may be of some help. Deeper tinea infections can be treated by an oral antifungal called griseofulvin; however, this is ineffective on candidiasis.

Viral infections

Three common viral infections are described here; herpes zoster, herpes simplex and warts.

Herpes zoster generally affects the adult population and is most commonly seen in those over 40 years of age.

Herpes simplex type I (see below) is found in virtually the whole adult population, although there may not be active signs (Baker, 1989).

Warts affect people of all ages.

Presentation

Herpes zoster (shingles) is characterized by an erythematous patch that quickly becomes oedematous, with groups of vesicles that may crust if the disease is not treated. The thorax is the commonest site, but in the elderly the face is often affected.

Herpes simplex is characterized by redness and swelling of the mouth or genital area prior to the formation of a blister or even a superficial ulcer.

Warts are usually well-circumscribed areas of dry, hard skin, sometimes raised and sometimes flat. Warts are often seen on the hands, but may be seen on the face, knees and elbows. Plantar warts (verrucae) are seen on the feet, and genital warts in the genital area.

Causes

Herpes zoster, otherwise known as shingles, is caused by the *Varicella zoster* virus. This same virus causes chickenpox in childhood, and the virus remains latent in the body to reappear in the form of shingles. If an adult is not aware of having had chickenpox as a child and develops shingles, he or she must have had a sub-clinical attack of chickenpox when young.

Herpes simplex type I is responsible for infections on the face, neck or upper limbs, whereas type II lesions are responsible for genital infections and are usually sexually transmitted.

Warts are caused by various viruses; 45 different viruses have been identified as causing cutaneous or mucosal warts.

Symptoms

Herpes zoster lesions are preceded by pain in the area that is going to be affected. Because the virus affects the nerves, acute pain and numbness are common and there may be scarring and pigmentation following an attack. Lymphadenopathy is not uncommon. In those who are elderly and/or immunosuppressed the vesicles may become larger blisters, and it is possible for the lesions to become necrotic.

Herpes simplex usually settles spontaneously, but it is often accompanied by fever, malaise and lymphadenopathy. The blisters feel sore and uncomfortable.

Warts are not normally uncomfortable unless they are in an area where pressure is frequently applied, such as on the soles of the feet. They can be very awkward if they are on the hands or fingers, especially if they become large or numerous.

Treatment

Acyclovir (topically or orally) is the most common antiviral treatments for herpes simplex and zoster. Warts may be removed with over-the-counter preparations, most of which contain salicylic acid, which 'burns away' the thickened hard skin. Cryotherapy using liquid nitrogen is a more effective way of removing common warts.

Infestations

An infestation occurs when living creatures invade the body. These creatures are called mites or lice and, although small, can be seen under a microscope. The two most common types of infestation are scabies and head lice.

Scabies

Any one can be infested with scabies, although those who are immunologically compromised are probably at greater risk. Owing to the mode of transmission, those living in close contact with others are more likely to be affected – e.g. residents in nursing homes, or where a number of family members share the same bed.

Presentation

The scabies mite is about 0.3–0.4 mm long. The mites infest humans by the fertilized female burrowing into the skin to lay her eggs. These mature in 2–3 weeks, and are then capable of reproducing too. The burrows appear as tiny black dots with slightly scaly grey-white lines attached to them. It is most common to see them in the finger webs and flexures, and on nipples, ankles, wrists and feet. A scraping taken from the burrow may 'dig out' a mite or one of its eggs, which can be viewed under the microscope (Mocsny, 1990).

Causes
Scabies is transmitted by close physical contact between humans. The mite cannot live off the human body, although it may survive for short periods of time in bedding.

Symptoms
Scabies is very itchy, with the symptoms becoming worse at night. Although a lot of skin diseases are itchier at night there is a very marked difference in the level of itch in scabies, which helps with diagnosis. Because of the excessive itching scratching is a common problem, and this can lead to skin excoriation and infection.

CASE STUDY

Vera Ducklington, 90 years old, tells her district nurse that she has been itching very badly over the last week and that it seems to get worse at night. On inspection the burrows are visible and thus scabies is indicated. Skin scrapings confirm that there are active mites, and the GP prescribes a scabicidal lotion. The lotion needs to be applied from her neck downwards. Scabies does not affect the face or scalp in adults, although it can do in children. Vera must not wash whilst the lotion is in place. Once the treatment has finished (usually 48 hours and two applications later), Vera will need help to bath the lotion off and must then change all her clothes and bed linen, which can be washed in the normal way.

The other concern is the need to trace all those who have had close physical contact with Vera within the last month. (It can take up to 30 days for the first itchy symptoms to occur; Elgart, 1993). Treatment for contacts is by a single application of the scabicidal lotion, unless they have active symptoms. On investigation the only person who has had close physical contact with Vera is her daughter, and so she needs to be contacted and treated. Vera is very worried about the scabies and thinks that she is unclean. Explaining the fact that she probably picked it up during a stay in hospital and that it is not a reflection on her personal hygiene is important for reassurance.

Head lice (Pediculosis)
These affect mainly school children.

Presentation
The first signs of head lice might be black flecks on children's pillows or collars, which are the empty egg cases of the lice. The scalp may be itchy, but the most common way of determining that lice are present is by seeing the greyish-white eggs attached to the hair shaft.

Cause
Head lice are spread by close contact between people, which is why school children are particularly prone to them.

Symptoms
Itchiness of the scalp is the most common symptom.

CASE STUDY

A mother brings her 8-year-old, Joe, to see the school nurse, describing black flecks on his collar. The most likely cause is that the child has head lice. The school nurse can see the eggs attached to the hair shaft. As there have been a number of other children with head lice in the school already this summer, another case comes as no surprise. Joe says that his head feels very itchy; he feels a bit embarrassed about it but knows that his best friend has just had head lice and so is not that worried.

The school nurse explains that the mother has two options. First, she can use an insecticide in the form of a lotion applied to dry hair. There have in the past been concerns about the safety of some of these lotions for children, although these concerns have not been conclusively proven (Butler, 1998). A single application of the lotion followed by a second one a week later should be sufficient. The second choice available to the mother is to wet-comb her children s hair using a fine-toothed nit comb and conditioner on the hair; this will physically remove the eggs from the hair shafts (the conditioner makes the hair slippery so that the eggs are removed more easily). This treatment takes longer, requiring a thorough combing every 3 4 days over a 2-week period (Butler, 1998).

Joe s mother knows that he will not sit still long enough to have lots of combing sessions, and therefore opts for the insecticidal lotion. As they leave with the lotion, the nurse reminds her to follow the instructions carefully and to continue to check her children s hair regularly. She also reminds Joe to tell his Mum if his head gets itchy again, and points out that there have been cases of resistance to the insecticides so vigilance about it s efficacy is important.

Conclusion

Although this chapter has only covered the tip of the iceberg, it has illustrated that there are many ways in which the skin can fail. Support and reassurance for patients cannot be overemphasized. Skin failure can lead to a patient feeling stigmatized and embarrassed, and it is important to remember that the psychological support offered by a nurse is as important as good physical care.

Reflective activities

1. Think about the sort of medical problems that patients on your ward have. Do any of them have an impact on the skin? If so, make a note of these and discuss with your colleagues how you can ensure that you meet the care needs of these patients.
2. Consider the last time you had a mosquito bite, and remember how irritating it was. Try and envisage what this would be like if it were all over your body. Make a list of all the resources you have on the ward that you could use to help someone who was itching badly. What advice would you give to someone who was itching?
3. Look through the information leaflets that are available on the ward. Do you have any on skin diseases? Discuss with your colleagues whether increasing the number of information leaflets you have would be helpful. Contact the self-help groups and drug companies for further information.
4. Reflect on how a chronic skin disease such as psoriasis might impact on your life, and make a note of all the things that you do which would be affected.
5. Review the number of wound dressings that you have on the ward. Ask your colleagues if they know how they are used.
6. Try wearing a compression bandage for a few hours and reflect on how it feels and how it might feel for someone who has a leg ulcer.

References

Baker, H. (1989). *Clinical Dermatology*, 4th ed. Baillière Tindall.
Basler, D. E. (1991). Actinic keratosis and premalignant skin damage. *Dermatol. Nursing*, **3(1)**, 37–40.
Benbow, M. (1995). Intrinsic factors affecting the management of chronic wounds. *Br. J. Nursing*, **4(7)**, 407–10.

Bergstrom, N., Kemp, M. G., Allman, R. M. *et al.* (1994). *Pressure Ulcer Treatment: Clinical Practice Guidelines.* Quick Reference Guide for Clinicians No. 15. US Department of Health and Human Services, Public Health Service, Agency for Health Care Policy and Research.

Bernhard, J. D. (1991). Itching in the 90s. International Symposium on Itch: Basic and Clinical Aspects, Stockholm, Sweden, May 17–19. *J. Am. Acad. Dermatol.,* **24(2)**, 309–10.

Bridgett, C. (1996). Behavioural approaches to treating atopic eczema. *Health Visitor,* **69(7)**, 284–5.

Butler, M. (1998). A guide to nurse prescribing of insecticides and anthelmintics. *Nursing Times,* **94(22)**, 55–7.

Bysshe, J. (1996). Eczema: making an unpleasant condition more bearable. *Prof. Care Mother Child,* **6(3)**, 59–61.

Cameron, J., Wilson, C., Powell, S. *et al.* (1992). Contact dermatitis in leg ulcer patients. *Ostomy/Wound Management,* **38(9)**, 8–11.

Cooper, R. and Lawrence, C. (1996). The role of antimicrobial agents in wound care. *J. Wound Care,* **5(5)**, 374–80.

Cullum, N., Luker, K., McInnes, E. *et al.* (1998). *The Management of Patients with Venous Leg Ulcers: Technical Report.* Royal College of Nursing.

Dangel, R. B. (1986). Pruritus and cancer. *Oncol. Nursing Forum.* **13(1)**, 17–21.

David *et al.* (1983).

Dealey, C. (1994). *The Care of Wounds.* Blackwell Scientific Press.

Denman, S. T. (1986). A review of pruritus. *J. Am. Acad. Dermatol.,* **14(3)**, 375–92.

Donald, S. (1995). Atopic eczema: management and control. *Paed. Nursing,* **7(2)**, 29–35.

du Vivier, A. W. (1997). *Atlas of Clinical Dermatology,* 2nd edn. CV Mosby Co.

Elgart, M. L. (1993). Scabies: diagnosis and treatment. *Dermatol. Nursing,* **5(6)**, 464–7.

European Pressure Ulcer Advisory Panel. (1998). Pressure ulcer prevention guidelines. *EPUAP Rev.,* **1(1)**, 7–8.

Flanagan, M. (1994). Assessment criteria. *Nursing Times,* **90(35)**, 76–88.

Flanagan, M. (1997). Choosing pressure sore at risk assessment tools. *Prof. Nurse* (Suppl.), **12(6)**, S3–S7.

Fletcher, J. (1997). Update: wound cleansing. *Prof. Nurse,* **12(11)**, 793–6.

Gilleaudeau, P. and McClelland, P. B. (1994). Cyclosporine: a new therapeutic option for severe, recalcitrant psoriasis. *Dermatol. Nursing,* **6(6)**, 395–407.

Graham-Brown, R. and Burns, T. (1990). *Lecture Notes in Dermatology.* Blackwell Scientific.

Hagermark, O. and Wahlgren, C. F. (1992). Some methods for evaluating clinical itch and their application for studying pathophysiological mechanisms. *J. Dermatol. Sci.,* **4(2)**, 55–62.

Hollinworth, H. and Kingston, J. E. (1998). Using a non-sterile technique in wound care. *Prof. Nurse,* **13(4)**, 226–69.

Kemp, M. G. (1994). Protecting the skin from moisture and irritants. *J. Gerontol. Nursing,* **20(9)**, 8–14.

Landis, E. (1930). Micro-injection studies of capillary blood pressure in human skin. *Heart,* **15**, 209–78.

Lawson, V., Lewis Jones, M. S., Finlay, A. Y., Reid, P., Owens, R. G. (1998). The family impact of childhood atopic dermatitis: the Dermatitis Family Impact Questionnaire. *Br. J. Dermatol.* 138, 107–13.

Le Lievre, S. (1996). Incontinence dermatitis. *Primary Health Care,* **6(4)**, 17–21.

Lock, P. M. (1980). The effects of temperature on mitotic activity at the edge of experimental wounds. In: *Proceedings of a Symposium in Wound Healing* (B. Sundell, ed.), Lindgren and Soner.

Mocsny, N. (1990). Care and treatment of scabies. *Adv. Clin. Care*, **5(5)**, 23–6.

Morison, M. (1994). *A Colour Guide to the Assessment and Management of Leg Ulcers*, 2nd edn. CV Mosby Co.

Nicole, N. H. and Fenske, N. A. (1993). Photodamage: cause, clinical manifestations and prevention. *Dermatol. Nursing*, **5(4)**, 263–77, 326.

Noren, P. and Melin, L. (1989). The effect of combined topical steroids and habit-reversal treatment in patient with atopic dermatitis. *Br. J. Dermatol.*, **121(3)**, 359–66.

Oliver, L. (1997). Wound cleansing. *Nursing Standard*, **11(20)**, 47–51.

Penzer, R. (1994). Helping patients to cope with psoriasis. *Nursing Standard*, **8(49)**, 25–8.

Perkins, P. (1996). The management of eczema in adults. *Nursing Standard*, **10(35)**, 49–53.

Phillips, J. (1997). *Pressure Sores*. Churchill Livingstone.

Plotnick, H. (1990). Evaluation work relevancy of dermatitis: basic cognitive skills. *AAOHN J.*, **38(11)**, 524–30.

Rich, A. (2001). How to … perform a Doppler ultrasound test. *Br. J. Dermatol. Nursing*, **5(2)**, 12–13.

Royal College of Nursing. (2001). *Pressure Ulcer Risk Assessment and Prevention*. RCN.

Savin, J. (1995). The measurement of scratching. *Sem. Dermatol.*, **14(4)**, 285–9.

Savin, J. (1998). The war against antibiotic resistance. *Dermatol. Practice*, **6(5)**, 4.

Scales, J. T. (1990). Pathogenesis of pressure sores. In: *Pressure Sores – Clinical Practice and Scientific Approach* (D. L. Bader, ed.), Macmillan Press.

Shmunes, E. and Keil, J. E. (1984). The role of atopy in occupational dermatoses. *Contact Dermatitis*, **11**, 174–8.

Somma, S. and Glassman, D. (1991). Malignant melanoma. *Dermatol. Nursing*, **3(2)**, 93–9.

Stewart, L. A., Engelken, G. J. and Nicol, N. H. (1992). Essentials of occupational contact dermatitis. *Dermatol. Nursing*, **4(3)**, 175–83.

Swartz, S. M. and Sherertz, E. F. (1993). The technique of patch testing: role of the office staff. *Dermatol. Nursing*, **5(2)**, 133–144.

Thomas, S., Jones, M. and Andrews, A. (1997). Special focus: tissue viability. The use of fly larvae in the treatment of wounds. *Nursing Standard*, **12(12)**, 54–9.

Thomlinson, D. (1987). To clean or not to clean? *Nursing Times*, **83(47)**, 71–5.

Torrance, C. (1983). Pressure Sores: Aetiology, Treatment and Prevention. Croom Helm, London.

Townsend, M. (1994). Just a glove? *Br. J. Theatre Nursing*, **4(5)**, 9–10.

van der Weyden, R. (1990). Basal cell carcinoma classifications and characteristics. *Dermatol. Nursing*, **2(4)**, 209–14.

Wahlgren, C. F. (1992). Pathophysiology of itching in urticaria and atopic dermatitis. *Allergy*, **47(2)**, 65–75.

Waterlow, J. (1987). Calculating the risk. *Nursing Times*, **83(39)**, 58–60.

Wilson, C., Cameron, J., Powell, S. *et al.* (1991). High incidence of dermatitis in leg ulcer patients: implications for management. *Clin. Exp. Dermatol.*, **16(4)**, 250–53.

Williams, C. (1991). Comparing Norton and Medley. *Nursing Times*, **89(36)**, 66–8.

Wright, A. (2000). London Review – an assessment of clinical evidence supporting the efficacy and safety of lanolin. St Luke's Hospital, Bradford.

Altered body image related to skin impairment

Su Bullus

Introduction

In a media-oriented society, the impression is created that in order to be loved, desirable and successful it is necessary to be thin, youthful and attractive, with a clear and unblemished skin. The skin therefore plays an important role as an organ of display, affecting the way a person's body is viewed by the rest of society. The impact of this role is particularly noticeable when patients have a visible skin impairment, as in those conditions that affect the face, neck and hands. It is useful to note, however, that an alteration in body image can also stem from less obvious disfigurement. Wright (1986) noted that a change in appearance anywhere in the body can produce an altered body image. Those suffering from both acute and chronic skin disorders, whether hidden or visible, can therefore experience a diminished body image.

Despite some acknowledgement that dermatology is a clinical area where body image is a problem (Price, 1986; Hitchens and Creevy, 1988), there is a surprising scarcity of research-based literature directly related to body image and skin disorders. Much of the existing literature is therefore anecdotal in nature. It is necessary, then, to apply the available information in a way that is relevant for patients suffering from skin disorders and can be utilized in a meaningful way.

Whilst nurses are becoming more aware of the potential problems of an altered body image, it is often the case that their ability to deal with this problem is limited. Although the reasons for this are complex, for example due to negative attitudes or a lack of skills and knowledge base (Mellor, 1996), it is reasonable to suggest that a growing awareness of this problem can promote an improvement of nursing skills in this important area of care. Whilst there are specialist areas dedicated towards caring for those with dermatological conditions, there are also many patients in all areas of health care who will be experiencing problems related to their skin, even if their skin is not their primary medical problem. The impact of what may seem a relatively minor problem is in some measure substantiated by a study of patients suffering from psoriasis. Ramsay and O'Reagan (1988) concluded that the emotional perceptions of this condition were just as prevalent in those patients with mild disease as in those with extensive disease. It is hoped that through reading this chapter healthcare professionals working in all areas will be able to develop insight into these potential problems in order to care for these patients more sensitively and effectively.

Body image

It is important to acknowledge that our body image is something that develops from birth and that stays with us for a lifetime. It is also important to realize that it changes at different times in our lives, both in health and in illness. It is essential to point this out because often body image is commonly regarded as something that afflicts us in much the same way as an illness, rather than as something that is a normal part of our being.

The longitudinal, perpetual and ever-changing phenomenon of body image is therefore totally individual and consequently difficult to define. One of the intrinsic difficulties in defining the term body image is that it is a complex and fairly abstract concept that has no absolute interpretation. This difficulty can be partly attributed to the fact that the term body image is a composite of both physiological and psychological factors (Janelli, 1986). It has been conceptualized by Schilder (1935) as 'the picture of our body which we form in our mind' – that is to say, the way in which our body appears to ourselves. Wood (1975) simplifies this definition further by describing body image as a mental picture of one's own body.

It has been suggested by Price (1990a) that there are three components that are all essential for the construction and maintenance of a normal body image:

1. Body reality, which refers to the way in which our body is constructed – the way it really is
2. Body ideal, which refers to the way we think that our body should look and act
3. Body presentation, which refers to how we present our body to the world through our dress, our pose or our actions.

In summary, then, body image is a composite of these three components and can be defined as the picture in our mind that we have of our body.

A further difficulty in attempting to define the concept of body image is that there are other concepts which, whilst related to body image, are not synonymous with it. Two of these are the relevant concepts of self-image and stigma. These concepts need to be examined in order to have an understanding of the psychological impact of an altered body image.

Self-image

Whilst body image can be defined as the mental picture of the body, self-image refers to the mental picture of the total personality. Body image is therefore just one part of this total personality (Bailey and Clarke, 1989). Price (1990a) suggests that our self-image is constructed from two parts; one aspect is formed by our personality, and the other part is the social self created by socialization into the world. Socialization begins at birth and continues throughout life. It can be defined as the process by which we learn the ways of thought and behaviour that are considered appropriate to a society. Social characteristics are then acquired that enable the individual to be accepted within a particular society. An example of this is the teenager who starts smoking because others in the peer group also smoke.

Umiker (1993) supports the view of Price (1990b) by suggesting that self-image is formed from a multiplicity of facets. These facets include both parental expectation and the expectation of ourselves and others. Self-image is a reflection of how we have been treated by others and also how we compare ourselves to others, although parental treatment is the most important (Umiker, 1993). Price (1990b) explains the importance of body image to the formation of self-image by suggesting that a healthy body image is an essential attribute for the enhancement of self-image (see Figure 4.1). Alternatively explained, it could be said that how we feel about ourselves is related to how we feel about our bodies. Body image can therefore play a vital part in self-understanding (Bycroft, 1994). This is relevant for those with a skin impairment, because a skin impairment can cause psychological disturbance and a lowering of self-image (Schuster, 1991).

Stigma

An alteration in body image and the subsequent damage to self-image can be linked to the concept of stigma. Stigma has been

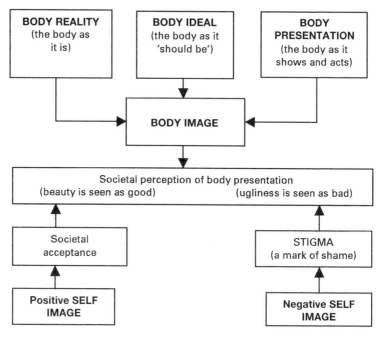

Figure 4.1 The relationship between body image, self-image and stigma.

simply defined as a mark of shame (Saylor, 1990). This seems to be a particularly pertinent description when considering stigma associated with skin impairment. Goffman (1963), however, maintained that stigma is not just a mark of shame but also the response that society makes towards this mark, and asserted that stigma occurs when a person's appearance and social identity poses a threat to society's concept of normality.

Patients with a skin impairment are often stigmatized by feeling shunned by other people, and that they are less welcome in society. This is important to consider when caring for patients with any degree of skin impairment. The experience of simply being a patient in any healthcare setting can cause anxiety and a change in bodily perception, and a skin impairment and the subsequent alteration in body image and self-image can increase the anxiety. If health professionals themselves portray a negative attitude towards the patient, however unwittingly, the problem may become compounded. Stigma is, after all, a social creation, and the world of health care is another social situation for the individual to meet.

It is therefore useful to identify the link between the concepts of body image, self-image and stigma, because an individual with a skin impairment may become stigmatized by society. This stigma may produce an altered body image, which in turn could result in a poor self-image.

Development of body image

Our body image is said to change and develop throughout life (Price, 1990b), and this development often occurs at the significant stages of life, such as puberty, pregnancy, menopause and ageing. Whilst these developments are dynamic, they are merely recognizable stages in the normal development of body image.

Body image changes appear to become differentiated in early life when a child learns to become separate from the parents. The child psychologist Piaget (1958) indicated that an infant has no body image at birth because body image is developed alongside psychological, social and physiological development. A child will perpetually integrate experiences from the world and develop responses to this world. Thus the development of body image in a child is a learned phenomenon, and a child is constantly redefining a body image perception. Darbyshire (1986) comments that parental perceptions about whether their baby is likeable and clever are related to the physical attractiveness of the baby. The child's body image is therefore closely related to the positive or negative attitudes of parents, and thus a child with a skin impairment can potentially suffer from the negative perceptions of others even at an early age. This is exemplified by parents who have described how their children seem less popular than other children. They may have less interaction with other children because the children and their parents are wary of a child with a skin impairment.

This body image change becomes intensified towards puberty, when there are great physical and psychological changes. The profound changes in normal body image development during adolescence are accompanied in many instances by a desire to fit in with peer groups. Cronan (1993) describes this as the desire to conform with group norms. It could be argued then that an alteration of body image might have more of an impact at this significant life stage. Even small blemishes can be socially and emotionally debilitating during adolescence, and MacKie (1991) declares that the psychological impact of skin impairment can be greater during a significant period in development such as adolescence. This in itself highlights the particular problems of the adolescent. It has already been suggested that anyone with an alteration in body image is seen as deviant from the norm, and this could mean that a person suffering from a skin disorder will not be accepted by the group or indeed will shy away from the group altogether. Many adolescents cite difficulties in going to public places, such as the swimming baths, where most of the body is exposed. The adolescents become conscious that others are staring at them, and this has a particularly negative impact at a time when adolescents are trying to 'fit in' with the group.

These important periods of development where a skin impairment has a significant impact are not confined to childhood and adolescence. After the period of adolescence, body image continues to alter with the bodily changes associated with ageing. The older, mature individual is one who has integrated all bodily experience successfully (Bailey and Clarke, 1989) and has learned to accept his or her body image. Whilst body image develops further with this ageing process, the changes associated with ageing may have a great psychological impact in some people. In part this can be attributed to the fact that western culture places its emphasis on youth, attractiveness and wholeness, and thus the potential for an altered body image can also increase with age. Janelli (1993) states that this is because the elderly are more susceptible to illness, and therefore an associated alteration in body image can become more common.

The final stage in body image development is at the approach of death. Cronan (1993) states that just prior to death body image is consolidated either with dignity or neglect, and attention to appearance can greatly enhance the dignity of the patient. In this final stage of life, body presentation becomes of vital importance to body image consolidation. Family, friends and of course nurses may have to fulfil this role where the patient is not able to in the final phase of body image formation.

In summary, the development of body image is a normal process within the boundary of all human development throughout the life cycle.

Body image as a social construct

Society plays a large part in the formation of body image (Salter, 1988). The value of our body is negotiated in every social encounter (Price, 1990b), and so body image is often viewed as a social creation (Drench, 1994). As already stated, society values attractiveness, and a plethora of studies show that, in a wide range of social situations, the physically attractive are the most favoured (Newell, 1991). The mass media reinforce this stereotype by consistently implying that it is necessary to have a pleasant, healthy appearance (MacGinley, 1993). Society can dictate what is normal, and this view of normality is accepted by many people. The result is that society can exert pressure on an individual to comply with this certain image. It seems necessary to have a normal appearance in order to gain social acceptance and approval.

It is also through social interaction that an individual learns the habits of a particular culture that are related to body image. Culture can be described as the values, norms, practices and beliefs of any group that guide thinking and action. Body image becomes culturally bound because all world cultures have their own perception of body image. The body image of each individual is therefore measured against a cultural standard. What is considered normal in one culture may not be the case in another – in western culture thinness is valued, whereas in certain African tribes a neck stretched by brass rings is considered desirable. The nurse needs to be cognizant with these differences, but also to recognize that an unblemished and smooth skin has been considered a commonality across all cultures (Fallon, 1990). It can be predicted, however, that there will be greater uniformity of cultural standards in the future with the expansion of the mass media.

The issue of gender is another important factor in the social construction of body image. This is especially relevant when considering the visibility of a skin impairment. A review of the literature suggests that the influence of body image on self-image is greater for women than for men. Women appear to be much more concerned with their body appearance (Price, 1993), and women are more likely than men to equate self-worth with their own attractiveness. Conversely, a man's self-image is more related to fitness than appearance. McBride (1988) confirms the social construct of this view by proposing that whatever constitutes beauty at a particular age in time is what women aspire to attain during that period. Rubens, who painted in the seventeenth century, has recorded this change in perception. He painted large, fleshy women, who were considered attractive at that time. Even in the seventeenth century, though, all the women he painted had perfect, unblemished skin.

It becomes apparent then that not only does the social world help to shape our body image; our body image also has a fundamental effect on our social lives. There is evidence that indicates that those suffering from a skin impairment seriously curtail their social activity due to the negative reaction of the general public (Ramsay and O'Reagan, 1988). In this study, the individuals with a skin impairment felt that the public were staring at them and also seemed to have a limited knowledge and understanding of skin impairments. To illustrate this point, a patient recently cited an instance where the cashier at the local chemist always dropped change into the purse or the palm of the lady's hand without touching her because she has severe hand scarring. This individual now makes a much longer journey to another chemist where the cashier does not react in this way.

It is pertinent for nurses to be aware of the literature that indicates that the appearance and attractiveness of patients can affect the attitude of nurses as well as the public (Nordholm, 1980). Appearance has been shown to have a strong influence on relationships, where the physically attractive are viewed in a more positive way than those who are less attractive (Darbyshire, 1986). It is important, then, that nurses are aware of any personal bias that they may have, as negative attitudes could have a detrimental affect on the patient's body image.

It is clear that the attitude of an individual, and indeed of society as a whole, may produce a negative body image and therefore a diminished self-image in a person suffering from skin disease.

Reactions to change in body image

Whilst body image is a changing concept throughout human development, an altered body image is not part of this normal process. An altered body image is, therefore, a negative experience, which MacKie (1991) describes as a change outside the boundary of human development. An altered body image is said to occur when there is a failure to accept the body as it is, and an alteration of body image may occur at any stage throughout the life cycle (Price, 1990a). It is important to recognize this, as a skin impairment can also span all age groups and the psychological impact of a skin impairment may depend upon these critical periods in development.

An alteration of body image may affect people in different ways, and so body image can be seen as an important determinant of behaviour (Model, 1990). The effect of an alteration in body image will also depend on factors already discussed, such as age, gender or cultural background. These reactions are said to be related to the nature of the alteration and how significant it is for the person suffering from it (Drench, 1994). The significance of this alteration in body image therefore depends on the person experiencing it and on whether they perceive this to be a negative alteration.

There are several emotions that an individual may experience as a result of an alteration in body image. These emotions include fear, shame, hopelessness, anxiety and depression (Bailey and Clarke, 1989). There are several theoretical models that can be examined in order to identify possible reactions to an alteration in body image.

Nurses are now familiar with the widely accepted stages of grief model devised by Kubler Ross (1969). Whilst this model has been extensively used to enlighten care for the dying, there are many parallels to be drawn with those suffering from the loss of an accepted body image. The surmise is that those with an altered body image will also go through a grieving process. This process constitutes six stages:

1. Shock
2. Denial
3. Anger
4. Depression
5. Bargaining
6. Acceptance.

Price (1990a) remarks that the progression through these stages is not necessarily sequential, and there may be a return to the earlier grief stages. Price (1990a) also states that the final acceptance stage may take a considerable amount of time to reach or indeed may never be reached. MacGinley (1993) also suggests that the patient will hopefully progress through these stages, but in no particular set order. It may be that these views are identifiable depending upon the individual grief reaction of each patient. This model does therefore seem to be useful in enabling nurses to recognize possible reactions to an altered body image.

In comparison, Dewing (1989) has suggested that there are four stages of adjustment to an altered body image:

1. Impact, when the individual recognizes the change
2. Retreat, when the individual withdraws from the change
3. Acknowledgement, when the individual faces the change
4. Reconstruction, when there is a reorganization of lifestyle.

The stages of grief model (Kubler Ross, 1969) and Dewing's (1989) stages of adjustment appear to have much in common.

Whilst 'shock' and 'impact' have similar connotations, shock implies a more negative emotion. As Price (1990a) asserts, there may be some individuals for whom an alteration in body image is not undesirable – for example, where taking on patient status relieves an individual from normal responsibilities. A skin impairment may then be an advantage for that person, and 'impact' may be a more useful term to use.

Ultimately an individual may never reach the stage of 'acceptance', and perhaps for certain individuals 'acknowledgement' may be a more realistic aim. The Dewing (1989) model, however, considers that 'reconstruction' is the final stage. This stage concerns a reorganization of lifestyle, but perhaps this is not always the ultimate stage for every individual. In certain circumstances those with a skin impairment need to be able to keep their lifestyle the same – for example, continuing to go swimming despite the skin impairment. This may mean that acceptance is again the most useful goal.

These possible grief reactions to an alteration in body image can be seen as coping strategies. Bailey and Clarke (1989) describe three commonly used coping strategies:

1. Direct coping, involves the patient being able to rationalize the alteration in body image in the same way as other people not directly involved in the situation may do. Successful direct coping should therefore result in reduced stress.
2. Indirect coping, is used when the patient feels unable or unwilling to accept the alteration in body image. This means that the patient has to change his or her perception of the alteration in body image, and that subsequently nurses' and patients' perception of the same body image change may be very different.
3. Palliative coping, which is action that relieves immediate stress without helping the problem. Examples include drinking alcohol to excess, or over-eating.

Palliative coping and indirect coping do not lead to a long-term acceptance of the alteration in body image. Both these coping mechanisms may relieve stress but will not result in sustained coping with the alteration in body image.

Evidence of these grief reactions and coping strategies can be seen in the following example.

It could be argued that Ben was showing a typical grief reaction by retreating from his problems and becoming depressed about them. Closeting himself away from the world was merely a palliative strategy that was not attempting to deal with the problem of an altered body image. Ben had not worked his way through the whole process of grieving as identified by Kubler

> **Example**
> Ben was an 18-year-old man who had been suffering from psoriasis for 14 months. The main areas affected were his scalp, hairline, hands and arms. Because of the visibility of the problem Ben had become reclusive, leaving the confines of his home only to visit the local hospital. He could no longer tolerate any public situation, and even avoided his closest friends. The avoidance of all contact with others had stopped him attending the local technical college. He had therefore not obtained the qualifications he wanted, and was unemployed. He was ashamed of his appearance and had become very withdrawn and depressed.

Ross (1969) and Dewing (1989). Help from healthcare professionals may well have meant that progress forward could be made.

It has been suggested that whatever phases or stages may be recognized as the reaction to an altered body image, adaptation can only begin when the individual can acknowledge this change (Bailey and Clarke, 1989). It is important for nurses working in all healthcare settings to be able to recognize altered body image when it has happened, as well as the possible reactions to the change. In conclusion, the response to an alteration in body image is highly individual and complex.

Applying theory to practice

The nurse is in a unique position to help patients re-establish a body image that is acceptable to them. The reasons for this include the nurse's close and continuous proximity to the patient, the intimate nature of nursing, the opportunity to explore patients' private fears and concerns, and the ability to advance a holistic approach to care. Once it has been established that a patient with a skin impairment is suffering from an altered body image, a realistic nursing plan of care needs to be formulated. Price (1990b) suggests a model for body image care that clearly sets out five modes of care intervention:

1. Preventive care
2. Supportive care
3. Patient education
4. Patient counselling
5. Liaison with support networks.

The first care mode identified by Price (1990b) is that of preventative action. This pre-emptive action is to ensure that an alteration of body image does not occur. Whilst many types of skin impairment may be unavoidable, for example following a chronic skin condition, there are actions that can be taken to try to lessen the environmental affects that may result in a body image impairment. An example of these is sun avoidance and use of sunscreens to lessen the effects of ageing, burning or skin cancer. Other health promotional issues, such as avoidance of accidents in the home to prevent burns, would also be relevant to this mode of care and the domain of skin impairment. Whilst important, the preventive mode does not actually inform clinical practice to assist those who already have a skin impairment.

The supportive care mode does assist the patient who is already experiencing a body image impairment. Price (1990b) indicates that supportive care relates to physical ways of improving body image perception. This could mean helping a patient to dress in such a way that would disguise the skin impairment, or changing a wound dressing for a clean one. This could be especially useful where a patient has a particularly malodorous wound such a fungating breast tumour or a leg ulcer. The issue of privacy is also crucial within the supportive care mode. There is greatly reduced privacy in the hospital setting, and healthcare professionals have a duty to protect the dignity and privacy of those in their care (Thompson *et al.*, 1988). Privacy is not just a matter of avoiding exposure, it is also a notion about patient vulnerability (Lawler, 1991). The patient with a body image impairment is in a vulnerable state, and as such needs the provision of privacy in a civilized and caring manner.

Education is seen by Price (1990b) as the way in which patients can regain control of their healthcare. Nurses also need to be able to educate the patient's family about altered body image because their involvement can provide continuing support for the patient at home, and education can help to ensure that the patient's perception of his or her body image is not devalued by them. For example, families may be exasperated by teenagers who feel that a skin impairment is socially devastating because from their point of view it seems physically so insignificant. The nurse can help to facilitate an understanding about this problem through education and explanation.

Counselling is deemed to be crucial for the patient who is undergoing a grief process, and Kelly and Henry (1992) suggest that early counselling following diagnosis is especially useful for these patients prior to surgery. This may be especially relevant to those who may face a loss of skin integrity and subsequent skin impairment following their surgery. The role of the nurse is to reassure the patient that the spectrum of emotions experienced is normal. Staff should be aware that patients need the opportunity to discuss feelings, and be prepared to listen to these (Bailey and Clarke, 1989). However, Mellor (1996) qualifies this assertion by reminding nurses that what patients hear and what is being said to them may be different. Nurses therefore need to provide realistic encouragement, stressing an individual's positive strengths. The key to a therapeutic reciprocity is the non-judgemental attitude of the nurse and the acceptance of the patient's feelings and viewpoint. This can help the patient to move towards the acceptance of an altered body image.

Price (1990b) suggests that part of the role of the nurse is liaison with support networks. This is because it is of crucial importance to all healthcare professionals that how patients accept an illness is related to the attitude and behaviour of those around them (Schilder, 1989). Leonard (1972) remarks that the reaction of family and friends towards a physical impairment can markedly influence adaptation towards an altered body image. As the most significant care provider, the nurse needs to understand the importance of the family in the overall plan to help the individual cope. Kelly and Henry (1992) have suggested that partners in particular have in the past received insufficient counselling. Patients with an active social support network are more likely to come to terms with an alteration in body image. MacGinley (1993) recommends that nurses need to recognize the importance of these support networks so that they can be utilized to help the patient's adjustment to an altered body image.

The nurse's role in caring for those with an altered body image has also been usefully and succinctly described by Dewing (1989), and nine types of support identified within that role:

1. Preoperative preparation and assessment planning
2. Provider of support and encouragement
3. Adviser
4. Non-critical listener
5. Care-giver
6. Educator
7. Co-ordinator and evaluator of care
8. Referral agent
9. Counsellor.

There are many similarities between this summary of the nurse's role and the modes of care intervention as described by Price (1990b). Dewing (1989) does, however, highlight the importance of three concepts to the nursing care of those with a body image disturbance: attitude, touch and normalization, which are discussed below.

Attitude

Dewing (1989) maintains that nurses need to adopt a positive attitude towards patients with an altered body image. The feelings of patients can be influenced by the nurses caring for them. Nurses' attitudes should be positive enough to help both the patient and the family to be sensitive to each others' needs (Cronan, 1993), without being unrealistic. Unfortunately nurses are not always aware that their attitude towards a particular patient can affect the care that they deliver (Leonard, 1972). This is especially pertinent to patients with a skin impairment who may already have experienced the negative attitudes of society attached to their condition.

Touch

Touch is an essential component of nursing care, and can help to reduce the stigma felt by many patients with a skin impairment. Mellor (1996) declares that every patient contact is significant because confidence may be enhanced or undermined in many ways. Touch can also be usefully employed as a nursing strategy to promote a positive attitude towards patients with a skin impairment. Avoidance of touch may send a message to the patient that the nurse dislikes that particular patient. Seaman (1982) suggests that touch can convey acceptance and caring, and this is especially important for those patients who may already have less physical contact with the people that they meet due to the condition of their skin. Touch can therefore be used by nurses to enhance self-image and reduce stigma.

Normalization

Dewing (1989) recognizes that those with an altered body image may be stigmatized and no longer feel 'normal'. This feeling of not being normal is allied to the grief reaction experienced by those suffering from an alteration of body image. Portraying a positive attitude towards the patient can promote a sense of normalization, and touch is just one means of portraying this positive attitude. Nurses can help to relieve these feelings of abnormality by other means – for example, encouraging the patient to choose and wear his or her own clothes can promote normality. Ryan (1987) remarks that cosmetics are important contributors to confidence in those with a skin impairment, and advocates the use of make-up and grooming. Nurses can help and support patients in this.

Dewing (1989) maintains that patients should have a gradual social exposure, which should ideally take place prior to discharge, and Cronan (1993) states that this normalization process is often neglected. If it is not possible to instigate this, then the nursing role can include education of the patient's friends and relatives so that they are equipped to provide support when the patient returns to the community. Darbyshire (1986) emphasized this by stressing the importance of nursing in providing a secure, empathetic environment where the patient can try out a new body image.

Nurses do need to be aware, however, that not all patients will make progress towards adaptation, and other professional help such as psychotherapy may be warranted. Mellor (1996) also asserts that it is part of the nursing role to ensure that patients have a realistic idea of what medicine and nursing can offer in their quest for normality. The essence of the nursing role is essentially the nature of the therapeutic relationship developed between the nurse and the patient. A plan of care needs to be based on this relationship, and strategies devised to ensure that this can continue outside the healthcare environment.

Conclusion

Body image can be defined as the way in which we see ourselves. A skin impairment can affect all age groups and can be seen in many areas of health care. Rather than being something that afflicts us, like a disease, our body image is with us all the time. Patients will react to a change in body image in several ways. If nurses are to give effective care, these reactions need to be both recognized and accepted, even if the skin impairment seems trivial. Nurses should closely examine the needs of patients in their care to determine whether any skin changes have caused an alteration in body image.

The implications for those suffering from a skin impairment appear to be particularly relevant to a discussion of the impact of altered body image. What may be regarded by others as a trivial skin impairment may have a profound affect on the way an individual perceives his or her own body image. The less physically attractive, which may mean those with any sort of skin impairment, may receive less in the way of positive reinforcement from society. This can therefore result in a decrease in self-image and loss of self-esteem (Newell, 1991). In order to help patients and families cope with an altered body image, the nurse needs to understand the possible reactions from society, the patient, and indeed nurses themselves. Nurses can have a major role in influencing the self-image of those with an altered body image due to a skin impairment. This awareness, knowledge and understanding can then provide a basis for sensitive and holistic care in all the areas of health care that patients with a skin impairment may find themselves in.

Reflective activities

1. How would you describe your own body image in the context of the points made in this chapter? Have there been any events in your life that have caused you to have an alteration in your body image?
2. Consider a patient under your care who may be experiencing a change in body image. Why is this change occurring? How is the patient and his or her family and friends responding to the change?
3. Look at the care plan of a patient who may have had a change in body image. What is there within the plan that may help guide your care of this patient? Does the care plan need re-writing in a more explicit way?
4. What are your own personal feelings about a person with a skin disease (e.g. eczema or psoriasis)? How do you think the body image of someone with a skin disease might be different from that of someone who has undergone abdominal surgery?
5. Think about how society shapes our views of body image. It is interesting to reflect on the conflicting images that bombard the public via media. Is it helpful when a celebrity 'admits' to having, for example, a skin disease or a colostomy?

References

Bailey, R. and Clarke, M. (1989). *Stress and Coping in Nursing*. Chapman and Hall.
Bycroft, L. (1994). Understanding body image. *J. Commun. Nursing*, **Jul**, 4–8.
Cronan, L. (1993). Management of the patient with altered body image. *Br. J. Nursing*, **2(5)**, 257–61.
Darbyshire, P. (1986). Body image – when the face doesn't fit. *Nursing Times*, **82(39)**, 28–30.
Dewing, J. (1989). Altered body image. *Surgical Nurse*, **2(4)**, 17–20.
Drench, M. E. (1994). Changes in body image secondary to disease and injury. *Senior Nurse*, **19(1)**, 31–6.

Fallon, A. (1990). Culture in the mirror: sociocultural determinants of body image. In: *Body Images. Development, Deviance and Change* (T. F. Cash and T. Prudinsky, eds), The Guildford Press.

Goffman, E. (1963). *Stigma: The Management of a Spoiled Identity*. Pelican.

Hitchens, S. and Creevy, J. (1988). In: *Altered Body Image* (M. Salter, ed.), John Wiley and Sons.

Janelli, L. M. (1986). The realities of body image. *J. Gerontol. Nursing*, **12(10)**, 23–7.

Janelli, L. M. (1993). Are there body image differences between older men and women? *W. J. Nursing Res.*, **15(3)**, 327–39.

Kelly, M. and Henry, T. (1992). A thirst for practical knowledge. *Prof. Nurse*, **7**, 351–4.

Kubler Ross, E. (1969). *On Death and Dying*. Tavistock Publications.

Lawler, J. (1991). *Behind the Screens. Nursing, Somology and the Problem of the Body*. Churchill Livingstone.

Leonard, B. J. (1972). Body image changes in chronic illness. *Nursing Clin. North Am.*, **7(4)**, 687–95.

MacGinley, K. J. (1993). Nursing care of the patient with altered body image. *Br. J. Nursing*, **2(2)**, 1098–2011.

MacKie, D. (1991). Psychological aspects of skin disease. *Practitioner*, **235**, 356–60.

McBride, A. B. (1988). Fat: a woman's issue in search of a holistic approach to treatment. *Holistic Nurse Pract.*, **3(1)**, 9–15.

Mellor, D. (1996). Altered body image. *Prof. Nurse*, **11(5)**, 296–8.

Model, G. (1990). A new image to accept: psychological aspects of stoma care. *Prof. Nurse*, **5**, 310–16.

Newell, R. (1991). Body image disturbance: cognitive behavioural formulation and intervention. *J. Adv. Nursing*, **16**, 1400–1405.

Nordholm, L. A. (1980). Beautiful patients are good patients: evidence for the physical attractiveness stereotype in first impressions of patients. *Soc. Sci. Med.*, **14(1)**, 81–3.

Piaget, J. (1958). *The Child's Construction of Reality*. Routledge & Kegan Paul.

Price, B. (1986). Keeping up appearances. *Nursing Times*, **82(40)**, 58–61.

Price, B. (1990a). *Body Image. Nursing Concepts and Care*. Prentice Hall.

Price B. (1990b). A model for body image care. *J. Adv. Nursing*, **15**, 585–93.

Price, B. (1993). Profiling the high-risk altered body image patient. *Senior Nurse*, **13(4)**, 17–21.

Ramsay, B. and O'Reagan, M. (1988). A survey of the social and psychological effects of psoriasis. *Br. J. Dermatol.*, **18**, 195–201.

Ryan, T. J. (1987). The handicap of skin disease. *Contemporary Dermatol.*, **Aug/Sep**, 26–31.

Salter, M. (1988). *Altered Body Image*. John Wiley and Sons.

Saylor, C. R. (1990). The management of stigma: redefinition and representation. *Holistic Nurse Pract.*, **5(1)**, 45–53.

Schilder, P. (1935). *The Image and Appearance of the Human Body*. Kegan Paul.

Schilder, E. (1989). Bodily perceptions and their influence on health. *Nursing Standard*, **4(13)**, 30–32.

Schuster, S. (1991). Depression of self-image by skin disease. *Acta Dermatol. Venereol.*, **156**, 53, 71.

Seaman, L. (1982). Affective nursing touch. *Geriatric Nursing*, **3(3)**, 162–4.

Thompson, I. E., Melia, K. M. and Boyd, K. M. (1998). *Nursing Ethics*. Churchill Livingstone.

Umiker, W. (1993). Optimism, self-image and self-esteem. *Health Care Supervisor*, **12(1)**, 23–8.

Wood, N. F. (1975). *Human Sexuality in Health and Illness*. CV Mosby & Co.

Wright, B. (1986). *Caring in Crisis*. Churchill Livingstone.

Caring for the skin at home

Rebecca Davis

Introduction

The aim of this chapter is to consider some of the challenges that face people with a skin problem when they care for themselves at home. Such people may suffer prejudice from the general public, which is more acutely felt when not in the protected environment of a hospital. Unfortunately the discrimination may come not only from the public but also from ill-informed healthcare professionals. The historical background to prejudice against skin disease is examined in this chapter. Therapies themselves can also make treatment at home difficult to manage, so it is crucial that people receive nursing care at home or in their health centre as well as in hospital. This chapter aims to give those carers in the community an insight into how skin care can be managed, as well as giving hospital nurses a feel for the problems patients face once they have been discharged from their care.

Historical and political perspective

People with skin problems often report suffering from social isolation and prejudice (Jowett and Ryan, 1985). This perhaps dates from the time when many skin diseases were associated with infectious, potentially life-threatening and disfiguring conditions, such as leprosy and the plague. Psoriasis was only formally dissociated from leprosy in the nineteenth century. Historically, therefore, other people's rejection of skin disease and those who suffer from it may stem from self-preservation, protecting themselves from illness. Although this protectionism is not necessary, the rejection appears to have continued into the twenty-first century. Many people continue to feel isolated and excluded from everyday activities; swimming, for example, can become a nightmare, with others staring and making comments. It is not unknown for people to be asked to leave swimming pools because of their skin. The fight against the perception of skin diseases being contagious is not helped by the fact that some dermatology beds are still housed in infectious diseases units.

Dermatology itself is often referred to as a 'Cinderella' speciality that does not attract the funds and public concern that other high profile specialities enjoy. Yet there are enormous numbers of patients who seek medical advice for dermatological problems. It has been found that 15 per cent of all general practitioner (GP) consultations are dermatological (Royal College of General Practitioners, 1995): Gawkrodger (1992) estimated that in a single year 1 per cent of the population is referred to a dermatologist for a skin opinion. This is only the tip of the iceberg, as there are many people with skin problems who never consult their doctor. Surveys have shown that although a quarter of the population have a skin problem that would benefit from medical attention, about 80 per cent of them do not seek help (Williams, 1997). Unfortunately neither GPs nor general nurses receive extensive training in dermatology, so despite the fact that there is significant morbidity due to skin disease, individuals may well come into contact with healthcare professionals who do not know how to help them manage their problem. This fact has been highlighted by the All Party Parliamentary Group on Skin (1998), which published a document discussing the needs for training amongst healthcare professionals who look after patients with skin disease.

Ruane-Morris (1995) surveyed hospital nurses' perceptions of dermatology patients, using a questionnaire. Sixty first- and second-level nurses were involved; 30 from a large teaching hospital and 30 from a district general hospital. Of the respondents, 20 per cent thought the specialty boring, 45 per cent felt that the patients would be best looked after in the community, and 90 per cent stated that dermatology patients came into hospital because they could not look after themselves. The study highlighted the lack of importance and status that is attributed to dermatology by the nursing profession. Without placements in dermatology areas during nurse training, the speciality will have difficulty changing this perception and will continue to have problems in recruiting interested staff.

When patients first consult a healthcare professional about a skin problem, it is crucial that the professional can provide them with accurate information. If this does not occur they may end up using the wrong treatments or using the right treatments wrongly, and this can lead to anger, confusion and depression at their lack of progress. This fact was highlighted in a paper reporting the results of a nurse-led psoriasis clinic (Penzer, 2000). Patients will also incur considerable expense if they have to pay for a number of prescriptions. If conventional therapies do not appear to be working, patients may turn to alternative or complementary ones; these may be helpful, but once again if not used properly can lead to considerable angst and may prove to be a waste of money. Lack of progress in improving the skin condition may also lead to unnecessary amounts of time off work. Quite clearly, therefore, the results of skin disease not only impact greatly on the individual and family, but can also have a significant effect on the economy through days lost off work.

As with all areas of the health service, politics have had a considerable impact on dermatology and the way that services are provided. There has been a significant move away from providing dermatology services through inpatient beds to more outpatient and community care. The number of dermatology beds across the country has fallen dramatically. For example, in London there were 185 designated dermatology beds in 1990; by June 1994 this figure had fallen to 58 (British Association of Dermatologists, 1994). In some cases the designated dermatology units have been replaced with allocated beds on medical wards.

This shift has had a number of repercussions. First, there are more dermatology patients being looked after by non-specialist nurses, so it is crucial that hospital and community nurses increase their knowledge of skin conditions and how they can be effectively managed. Secondly, it has meant that the exposure of new trainee doctors and nurses to dermatology patients may well be more limited, thus further reducing the pool of knowledge about skin disease and care.

On a positive note these changes have meant a greater focus on the provision of skin care in the community, which is where it is most needed. The vast majority of people with skin problems do not need hospital admission, but do need good care in their homes or in the GP's surgery. The challenge, therefore, is twofold: to ensure that patients have access to specialist services in hospital when their condition is rare, needs diagnosing or is difficult to treat; and for the rest of the time to have community healthcare professionals with the capacity to provide care that enables effective management of the patient's condition.

A number of models have been developed to cope with the needs of skin care patients in a more community-focused way. Examples of these models have been highlighted in a report entitled *Assessment of Best Practice for Dermatology Services in Primary Care* (Dermatological Care Working Group, 2001). Whilst these models differ in their detail, the overall objectives are generally the same; to provide better skin care services to patients in the community, and to ensure that hospitals receive referrals that are relevant.

The NHS Plan (DoH, 2000) acknowledged that waiting times in dermatology were particularly problematic. As a consequence of this, the 'Action on Dermatology' project was initiated. Whilst the primary objective of this project was to reduce waiting times, it led to investment in a number of locally-driven pilot schemes that looked at alternative and innovative ways of delivering care. Many of these are community-based, with nurses playing a major role in care delivery. So far, the results of these pilot schemes are not available.

It is impossible to consider all the possible models of community-based dermatology services here. However, there follow two examples of how nurses can make a major contribution to the provision of skin care services that meet the needs of individuals in the community.

Liaison nurses

The importance of liaison between primary and secondary care is increasingly recognized, resulting in expanding numbers of liaison nurse appointments across all specialities (Venables, 1995). The chronic nature of many skin problems and the amount of information that patients may require to care for themselves has led to the development of these posts to help provide continuity of care. The way these posts are organized depends on many factors – for example, other services available in the dermatology department, responsibilities in the job description, and the level of liaison already established between the community and the hospital. Each liaison nurse has a slightly different role, which is dependent on all these issues; however, the main themes are discussed below.

Community staff cover a wide number of specialties within their workload. Liaison nurses act as a resource for these staff by providing education, being available for joint visits, sometimes taking on patient care, or simply discussing a case over the telephone. They provide a crucial link between the expertise of a dermatology department and the community. Admissions to hospital may be prevented by a liaison nurse intervening early on in a patient's care. If patients can be taught how to manage their skin successfully at home it may prevent acute flare-ups that require repeated admissions to hospital. Liaison nurses can provide support for patients who are waiting for a bed to become vacant in hospital. It is also helpful if patients can have a link person in their care so that even if they are seen by a number of healthcare professionals there is one constant person. The liaison nurse can be this linchpin, providing continuity of care between the hospital and community, and further continuity once the patient returns to the community.

In some areas the liaison nurse may be viewed with suspicion, as community staff may feel that they are being criticized for not caring for a patient correctly or that their ability is being questioned. The liaison nurse should be seen as a quality addition to the team rather than a threat to staff, as there is a wealth of information that nurses and healthcare professionals can share and thus learn from each other.

Nurse-led clinics

Nurse-led clinics can exist within primary or secondary care. In primary care they have historically been established for chronic disease management or health education (e.g. a diabetes clinic or a family planning clinic). Community nurses (usually practice nurses) have developed expertise in a particular area to enable them to see patients independently, with the back-up of a GP if necessary.

Many of the common skin problems are chronic in nature and require long-term management. Patients with diseases such as eczema, psoriasis and acne need support and advice on a long-term basis, and these needs can be effectively met by an appropriately trained nurse. For all three conditions considerable support and advice are necessary, not only because of the complexities of treatment but also because of the psychological impact. A recent study has shown that attending a nurse-led clinic can lead to considerable improvements for patients with psoriasis (Penzer, 2000). Symptomatology and quality of life improved following three structured visits with a nurse, which included information giving, advice about treatment application and psychological support (Penzer, 2000).

One argument against establishing such clinics for people with skin disease is that there is insufficient demand in a single practice to make it worthwhile. The introduction of Primary Care Groups and Trusts has meant that such a nurse might be employed to provide a service for a whole group of GP practices rather than just one, and this often makes the post more financially viable. The move to increased levels of nurse prescribing will also affect the way that nurse-led clinics are run in the future.

Health and social policy are inextricably linked and, as demonstrated here, it is important that nurses are aware of issues so that they can challenge and influence policy to campaign for the highest quality of service for patients. The increase in the amount of dermatological care provided in the community should not be seen as a threat to secondary care providers. Instead, those involved in primary and secondary care should work together to establish the best possible services for the patients who use them. This discussion has shown how nurses have a huge role to play in the provision of these services and should make a significant contribution to the development of them. Advisers to politicians should be briefed on the issues that concern patient care and reminded how limited resources affect direct patient care. It is imperative that nurses are aware of the rights of their patients, how possible changes will affect their care, and how they can get assistance.

Looking after the skin at home

Managing skin disease in the community presents many challenges for patients and their carers. One of the keys to successful management is ensuring that patients apply treatments correctly. The next section explores the issue of compliance and whether this is the best word to use to describe whether patients stick to treatment regimes or not.

Compliance?

A dictionary definition of compliance tells us that it is a disposition to yield to others and suggests obedience (*Collins Concise Dictionary*). Van Onselen (1998) questions whether this is the sort of language that encourages healthy patient–nurse partnerships in care, and suggests that there are usually extremely good reasons why patients do not comply. She recommends that the word concordance be used instead of compliance, as this suggests being in harmonious agreement and is therefore a more appropriate way of describing a nurse–patient relationship. Concordance can be achieved by negotiating and agreeing treatments that fit into people's everyday lives and exploring what motivates or demotivates a patient as far as treating themselves is concerned.

It is not only nurses who recognize the importance of concordance. The Royal Pharmaceutical Society now has a website totally dedicated to this subject (www.concordance.org). In it they state that concordance '. . . is an agreement reached between a patient and a health care professional that respects the beliefs and wishes of the patient in determining whether, when and how medicines are taken'. They acknowledge that concordance will be enhanced by taking this stance. The government too recognizes the role that patients have to play in managing their own chronic conditions. In the 1999 White Paper *Saving Lives: Our Healthier Nation* (DoH, 1999) the government speaks of 'expert patients' who are empowered by having the knowledge and ability to manage their own conditions.

Thus most effective care is achieved by healthcare professionals working with patients rather than telling them what to do. For example, many of the treatments for chronic skin conditions rely on topical medications, some of which have a strong smell and/or stain. Before labelling a patient as non-compliant, healthcare professionals have a responsibility for finding out how useable their patient has found their topical preparations. A simple change from an ointment to a cream might be sufficient to ensure that a patient concords with treatment.

An example helps to illustrate why concordance can be difficult for patients. A patient who had just had a scalp treatment with the prescribed shampoo and topical treatment entered a small shop. The other customers commented that they could smell something strange and, thinking that the strong smell of tar was a fire, they all rushed outside to investigate. Whilst this is an extreme example of an experience that some patients go through, it helps to illustrate why not everyone wants to comply with treatments at home.

Patients may not concord with their treatments for a variety of reasons, and Davis and Fallowfield (1991) highlighted the following factors as important:

- The duration and complexity of treatments
- The costs to the patient in terms of behaviour change and restrictions
- The patient's understanding and retention of treatment information
- The treatment's perceived credibility and efficacy
- The vulnerability and severity of illness as perceived by the patient
- The level of support and encouragement given to patients
- Problems that are caused by the treatments themselves.

Treatment for skin disease includes all of these factors. The treatments are usually complex, with patients possibly using five or more creams to different parts of the body. A single treatment may take 1–2 hours and is likely to be needed twice daily, although, with individualized care planning, treatments do not need to take this long. Sensible advice about how to minimize treatment times and how to fit them into usual routines goes a long way towards maximizing concordance as well as improving quality of life. The treatment period may be indefinite, as chronic skin problems tend to come and go, so it is of even greater importance that patients develop routines that suit their lifestyles. Sackett and Snow (1979) noted that the rate of failure to follow long-term programmes in non-acute conditions was 50 per cent, and this became worse with time.

The concordance of patients is difficult to measure, although it is generally accepted to be a problem in dermatology. A simple method is to find out how many tubs or tubes of cream the patient uses in a week or a month. If a 500 g tub of emollient lasts for 3 months in someone with severe eczema, that person is not using sufficient emollient and is therefore are not concording with the prescribed regime. The result of this under-utilization of treatment is that the patient is not likely to see his or her condition improve. Once it has been established that a patient is not using the treatments, it is crucial to find out why. It may be due to a lack of understanding, lack of time or a dislike of the cream – for example, a strong-smelling treatment may inhibit partners from sleeping together, and a soap substitute may feel as if it does not clean the skin properly.

To improve 'compliance' (Niven's use of the word), Niven (1989) suggested a number of approaches. Patients need to understand instructions for use of their treatment as, even with the best of intentions, if they have misunderstood how to use their medications they will not be able to comply. Communication with patients needs to be friendly and open, and the healthcare professional must first establish the current level of understanding, along with any fears and misconceptions. Instructions should be devoid of medical jargon, and written information should be given to supplement the discussion. Time for questions and answers is crucial.

Socially isolated patients are less likely to concord because they do not have encouragement from people around them. This can lead to a downward spiral, as these patients are likely to experience worsening skin condition and thus remove themselves even further from social contacts. This can clearly be a really serious problem for some people who suffer with skin disease.

Concordance can be improved by providing simple and clear treatment regimes and, where possible, involving family and friends to help with the treatments and/or give the patient support in continuing to use them. Laffrey *et al.* (1996) showed that of a sample of psoriasis patients being treated in a day-care centre, those with social support had a shorter recovery time. Before a treatment plan is decided upon, all the alternatives should be explored. Once this has been done, details should be given regarding how medicaments should be applied, how to make the application easier (e.g. making sure the ointment is not cold), how long it will to work (including a review date), and the precautions that can be taken to protect the home and clothing (e.g. dark clothing and bed linen will help to disguise some of the staining).

To encourage children to concord, parents need to try to make the treatment time fun – for example by having bath toys for the child to play with whilst having a medicated bath. Pretending that the child is in a beauty salon may make applying a scalp treatment more fun.

Nurses are in a unique position within health care to be able to provide information for the patients and their families. The nurse who has a good understanding of how the treatments should be applied and who is able to build a trusting relationship with patients will be able to encourage discussion of problems that patients are experiencing. Listening to patients and their current coping mechanisms can lead to greater knowledge, which can be adapted to enhance those mechanisms further.

Using topical treatments at home

Prior to commencing treatment in the home, the patient must be warned of any adverse effects (both on themselves and on their homes). The bath oils can make the bath slippery, and medicated bath oils may stain the bath permanently so even after the treatment has been discontinued the bath may never appear clean again. Although bath oils are routinely prescribed, emollient shower gels are available for those who prefer to shower. Dithranol and tar are commonly used to treat psoriasis, the former leaves a purple stain and the latter a green/brown one on anything they come into contact with, including the skin. Some antibiotic creams stain bright yellow. Although emollients are colourless, they can leave greasy marks on furniture and clothing.

Thus when choosing the most appropriate treatment both nurse and patient must bear in mind the 'messiness' factor to ensure the best option is chosen. There are many topical treatments available for skin conditions, some of which are mentioned in Chapter 3. Here some guiding principles are given regarding aspects of topical treatments that people in the community often ask about.

Emollient and moisturizing therapies

For many dry skin conditions, emollient therapies provide the basis of the treatment. Emollient is the collective term for soap substitutes, bath oils, and moisturizing creams and ointments. The emollients need to be used regularly and will probably need to be applied even when no active disease is present, as patients are likely to continue having dry skin. Dry skin conditions include eczema and psoriasis. For concordance to be achieved, patients need to be able to choose the emollients that are acceptable to them. Encouraging patients to make their own choice of moisturizer is important, and this can be aided by giving them a number of samples of different moisturizers to try out. Some patients find they require two moisturizers, a lighter one for use during the day so that they can resume their work after application, and a greasier one for the night time.

Patients should be advised to carry their moisturizer with them during the day so that they can reapply it whenever their skin feels dry or irritated. Whilst this is sensible, they will not want to struggle around with a 500 g tub with a greasy top that ruins everything it comes into contact with. Pharmaceutical companies are more aware of providing convenient dispensers and are becoming more inventive with the packaging of products. Moisturizers are now available with pump dispensers and aerosol sprays as well as the old tubs and tubes.

If neat packaging is not available, a small amount of moisturizer can be decanted from a large tub into something smaller and more manageable. If this is done, the patient must be warned about control of infection and advised that the moisturizer must be decanted with an implement other than the hand – for example a clean spoon – and the smaller pot cleaned daily. If this is not done, the skin scales and any bacteria from the hand will stay in the tub of cream. Since the tub is a good environment for bacterial growth, the next time the patient uses the moisturizer it may be contaminated and could cause a skin infection.

Topical steroids

The use of topical steroid therapy is a difficult issue for patients. The increasing amount of lay information on the television and in the newspapers giving advice about the side effects of treatment can be confusing and sometimes inaccurate. It is difficult for patients to be asked to use topical steroids on themselves or their children when they have only heard about the problems that can be incurred and none of the benefits. Nurses need to be prepared to impart a level of information that will ensure confident use of the topical steroid. Often concern about the side effects of topical steroids is so great that the patient either under-uses the steroids or decides not to use the treatment at all. One of the most confusing issues is how much to use. Lack of information on how much to use can increase anxiety about whether the treatment is causing more harm than good.

Topical steroids are used to suppress inflammation (e.g. in eczema). The action of the steroid is to control the symptoms of the condition, and it will not provide a permanent cure. The steroids are classified into four groups based on their potency (i.e. how strong they are). Wright (1992) advocated a colour classification to illustrate levels of potency (Table 5.1), but it should be noted that these colours do not correspond to the colours on commercially produced tubes of topical steroid (e.g. a commercial dermovate tube has a brown flash of colour on it, not a red one). The colours can be useful reminders for patients trying to

Table 5.1 Colour classification of topical steroids

Potency	Colour classification	Examples of topical steroids
Very potent	Red	Dermovate, Nerisone forte, Halciderm
Potent	Orange	Locoid, Tidesilon, Betnovate, Adcortyl, Propaderm, Lotriderm, Diprosalic, Synalar, Metosyn, Nerisone
Moderately potent	Yellow	Betnovate R.D, Steidex, Haelan Synalar 1 : 4, Nystadermal, Ultarlanum
Moderately potent	Green	Eumovate, Alphaderm, Modrasone
Mild	Blue	Hydrocortisone 1%, 0.5%, Cobadex, Efcortelan, Hydrocotisyl, Dioderm, Mildisone

remember which is the most potent steroid – the strongest colour (red) represents the most potent steroid (e.g. dermovate).

Topical steriods do have potential side effects, but these are minimized if the correct treatment is used in an appropriate dosage. One difficulty for patients is that prescriptions may be marked 'apply sparingly' or 'apply as directed by doctor', and unfortunately these instructions do not provide the patient with the amount of information necessary for them to use the steroids with the confidence that the treatment will not be causing harm. The possible side effects of topical steroids, as documented in the *British National Formulary* (1998), include:

- Worsening and spreading of untreated infection
- Thinning of the skin, which may be restored over a period of time after stopping the steroids, although the original structure will never return
- Irreversible striae atrophicae (stretch marks) and telangiectasia (broken veins at the skin surface)
- Contact dermatitis
- Peri-oral dermatitis
- Acne at the site of application
- Mild depigmentation.

These side effects appear alarming, and without thorough discussion the patient may decide that the condition is not worth the risk. In reality, experiencing any of these side effects is relatively rare. It is extremely important to have a balanced discussion of the issues, explaining that the side effects are mostly seen in patients who have used potent and very potent steroids, usually in incorrect amounts, for too long or on the wrong part of the body. If used properly, topical steroids are safe and effective treatments for many skin conditions.

There are certain criteria that can be observed to reduce the potential side effects of topical steroids. The following list includes both those cited by Bowman (1994) and other indications:

1. Potent steroids should not be used on the face or flexures (skin folds) unless specifically advised. The skin in these areas tends to be thinner, and therefore the thinning effect of potent steroids can be visible very quickly if used.
2. Moisturizers may be sufficient to treat dry, inflamed skin. They should certainly be used in conjunction with topical steroid therapy and applied liberally to the skin prior to the application of the steroid (the amount of time this takes depends on the greasiness of the moisturizer; a cream will take 10–15 minutes and ointment 30 minutes to an hour). If the skin

is well moisturized, it will be easier to apply the steroid evenly to the affected area. If the steroid is applied first it tends to act as the moisturizer as well, and more is applied than is necessary.

3. As the inflammatory condition settles, the strength of steroid should be reduced. Topical steroids should be reduced in strength in the same way that systemic steroid therapy is. If the patient uses a potent or very potent steroid to control the condition and then stops treatment altogether once it appears to have settled, there is a risk of developing a 'rebound' of the condition. The steroids will have suppressed the symptoms, but when they are withdrawn the condition can return – often worse than when it originally appeared. The steroids must therefore be reduced with regard to strength (i.e. very potent to potent to moderately potent to mild) and then discontinued, with a period of 3–4 days at each strength if the condition is under control.

4. Repeat prescriptions of potent and very potent steroids should be avoided. It is important that when a patient is on a potent steroid the healthcare professionals involved in the care are aware of how much steroid is being used. As already discussed, using too little topical steroid can be detrimental to the patient's condition while too much can lead to all the problems associated with steroid over-use.

5. Combination therapy with an antifungal or bacterial cream may be necessary to combat low-grade infection. Patients with certain skin problems (e.g. eczema) tend to be more prone to skin infections. However, steroids can mask the infection, and therefore the skin should be assessed for signs of infection prior to commencing the treatment.

6. Under-treatment is as undesirable as over-treatment. Due to uncontrolled discomfort, the patient may suffer unnecessary trauma to the skin through scratching. Insufficient application of a topical steroid initially can mean that a patient needs to use a potent steroid for longer, as the proper benefit is not being given. In the long run this can mean that the patient ends up using a greater amount of topical steroid than if it were used correctly. In addition, once the condition has become worse it may be more difficult to bring back to a manageable level. The treatment required to do this may also be more potent than the steroid that was originally prescribed.

7. Steroid potency is increased by occlusion, such as with wet wraps and paste bandages. The absorption of steroids increases when occluded to the skin with a dressing or bandage, and this could increase the likelihood of side effects. It should be noted that occlusion should not be used on skin that is infected.

The quantity of topical steroid that can be used effectively and safely in 1 week is stated in the *British National Formulary* (1998), and the recommended amounts are shown in Table 5.2.

A simpler way of measuring the correct amount of topical steroid is by using the 'fingertip unit' (Long and Finlay, 1991). This is a useful guide because patients do not require any extra materials to be able to use the method effectively. The amount of cream or ointment coming from the nozzle of the tube and covering from the tip of the finger to the first joint crease is approximately 0.5 g. Different areas of the body have an allocated amount of steroid that it is advisable to use, and these quantities are different for children and adults (Figure 5.1).

Table 5.2 The quantity of topical steroid (in grams per week) that can be used safely

Area treated	Quantity of steroid cream or ointment that can be used safely (g/week)
Face and neck	15–30
Both hands	15–30
Scalp	15–30
Both arms	30–60
Both legs	100
Trunk	100
Groin and genitalia	15–30

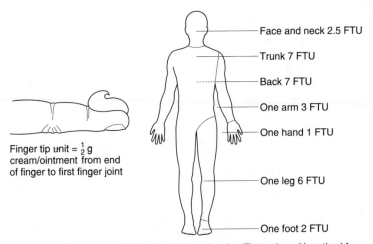

Finger tip unit = $\frac{1}{2}$ g cream/ointment from end of finger to first finger joint

Face and neck 2.5 FTU

Trunk 7 FTU

Back 7 FTU

One arm 3 FTU

One hand 1 FTU

One leg 6 FTU

One foot 2 FTU

Figure 5.1 Treatment guide for an adult, using the 'Fingertip unit' method for measuring topical steroid cream.

The use of the fingertip unit measurement guide should ensure the reduction of side effects due to incorrect dosage of the treatments. The fingertip unit is easily explained to patients, and provides them with the confidence necessary to continue treatments at home. To make life easier, the correct lengths of ointment or cream can be squeezed out prior to treatment. This means that during the treatment the tube does not have to be constantly squeezed with greasy hands.

Occlusive therapy

The care of children with atopic eczema is an area in which the family and the healthcare professional have to work closely together. It is crucial for the parents to be able to manage the eczema and encourage the child to have a relatively normal childhood that does not involve lengthy stays in hospital and time off school. The mainstay of eczema treatment is a combination of emollient and steroid use, and a good text for further detail is *Eczema and Your Child* (Mitchell *et al.*, 1998). In some cases these methods of treatment can be made more effective by occlusion – i.e. by covering up the skin once the treatments have been applied. Wet wraps are a common method of occlusion used in children with eczema. Their main indications for use are in an acute flare-up and/or when a child is particularly itchy and uncomfortable at night. Although it is possible to use wet wraps at other times, usually emollient alone or emollients and steroids are sufficient to keep the eczema under control.

If wet wrapping is appropriate, parents will need help to learn the technique and support in the early days of doing it. The key is to keep the technique simple. Usually the child has a bath using the prescribed bath emollient, and the skin is then patted dry. Afterwards the child has topical steroid applied to the affected areas. (The person applying the treatment should wear gloves to prevent unwanted contact with the topical steroid.) Moisturizers are then liberally applied all over, followed by the topical steroid. Because the moisturizer and steroid are going to be occluded they will sink in well, and therefore no wait is necessary between applying the treatments. As mentioned earlier, it is unusual to apply the topical steroid before the moisturizer, but in this case there is the need to get the wet wraps on as quickly as possible after the ointments have been applied. If the moisturizer were applied first and not allowed to sink in, the topical steroid applied over it would not be able to penetrate the large amounts of moisturizer and would 'slip off'.

Nine lengths of tubifast are then cut; two for each limb and one for the body. The width of the tubifast will depend on the size of the child, but generally green stripe is suitable for arms, blue for legs and yellow for the body. One length for each limb is put in warm water, wrung out well and then applied. Once each limb is covered with a wet layer, a dry layer should be put over the top of it. Only a dry layer is used on the trunk. All the parts are then tied together to hold them in place. Lawton has written an excellent guide to wet wrapping (Lawton, 1999).

The best time for wet wrapping is prior to the child going to bed. Being in bed tends to be when most itching and scratching occurs, and is therefore when the skin needs most protection. Because the wet wraps include a wet layer they can make the child feel cold, and it is therefore important that the child remains indoors after wet wrapping.

The treatment has provided great relief for both children and their parents. For some children one application can bring immediate relief, and they have their first good night's sleep in ages. For others, whilst the results are not as dramatic, gradual signs of improvement are seen. A specific example is the case of a toddler who had always resisted the topical treatments, screaming and wriggling to avoid applications. After a couple of days of wet wraps the child was quiet during the application and even offered her arm for treatment.

The treatment works by cooling the skin's inflammation, so hence calming the child and the irritation. If the child scratches the skin then one layer of tubifast is simply moved over the other, thereby reducing damage to the skin's surface. This allows the skin a chance to heal itself. The layer of damp tubifast over the moisturizer forms a seal over the skin, trapping the water in the epidermis and allowing rehydration. Once the skin is rehydrated, the sensation of irritation will be reduced. Note that, due to the occlusive moist nature of the treatment, it is not suitable for skin that is infected.

The frequency of treatment will vary from individual to individual, and it is important that it is appropriate for each child. This treatment needs considerable support from the nurses involved, but the benefit is that the parents usually feel that they achieve some control. Once parents feel they have this control their contact with the health service may dramatically decrease as they have the means to manage the eczema rather than allowing it to control the lives of their family. Many parents have expressed relief at feeling in control and being able to enjoy life again, some taking the opportunity to go on holiday now that they are no longer afraid of the eczema flaring up and not being able to cope.

Although wet wraps can be used on adults, they are not as successful. The same sort of occlusive effects can be gained by using paste bandages applied to limbs. Paste bandages tend to contract as they dry, and therefore need to be applied in such a way as not to create a tourniquet effect on a limb. They are applied using a pleating technique where, rather than winding the bandage round and round a limb, the bandage is folded backwards and forwards on itself. To keep these bandages in place tubifast can be used in a similar way as with wet wraps, or alternatively tubinette with bandages on top. The treatment is quite messy to apply and can restrict movement; patients often say that they feel a bit like Egyptian Mummies.

Other topical treatment

When choosing an appropriate topical therapy, one important consideration is the amount of time available to the individual. For example, short-contact dithranol is an effective treatment for plaque psoriasis. Although traditionally used in hospitals and day centres, now that an increasing number of patients are being cared for in the community this is a treatment being used by many at home. It involves a dithranol preparation (usually a cream) being applied to all the psoriatic plaques (except on the face). This is precise work, as dithranol will irritate the surrounding skin and must therefore be applied carefully just to the plaques. Hands should be washed immediately after application. The treatment is left on initially for a minimum of 20 minutes (this is then gradually increased as tolerance is achieved), and is then removed by the patient bathing or showering. It is obviously a time-consuming treatment.

Dithranol is just one of a number of treatments that are more suitable for use at home as the cream can be washed off reasonably quickly. The principle of all treatments is the same. The skin must be moisturized first and then topical treatments applied once this has soaked in.

A tremendous amount of discipline and motivation is required to commence this treatment every evening after a hard day's work, at a time when other people may be relaxing in front of the television or enjoying an evening out. Patients will require the support of family and friends to ensure that they have some success and remission. It is therefore important to include the patient and any significant others in the treatment choice and education so as to maximize support of the patient and success of the treatment.

Scalp treatments can cause great distress, as the treatments make the hair appear greasy, can colour the hair temporarily, often smell strongly, and stain bed clothes. A patient once joked that there should be a warning on the packaging that the commencement of treatment may initiate grounds for divorce. Despite some of the unpleasant side effects of scalp treatment, its application can be very relaxing as it is similar to receiving a scalp massage. The benefit of creating a relaxing time can help to reduce stress. The time can be used as quality time for a couple, who can spend the half-hour of treatment time talking together. If the treatment time is enjoyable for both people, the likelihood of concordance is increased.

Alternative therapies

Complementary therapies

The lack of cures for skin problems means that many patients turn in desperation to the vast number of advertisements offering relief from their condition. Whilst some of these make unfounded promises to vulnerable people, others do have some success. The attraction of these treatments is that they are often advertised as natural, which many people equate with safety; however, it must be pointed out that complementary therapies are not without potential side effects, and care must be taken when choosing them. They should be seen as complementary to rather than as alternatives to mainstream conventional therapies (Frost, 1994). The most commonly used complementary therapies in dermatology are Chinese herbal medicine and evening primrose oil.

Chinese herbal medicine involves the patient being assessed by a Chinese herbalist. The patient may be advised to alter his or her diet, and a herbal preparation will be prescribed. The preparation may be in the form of a tea or a cream. The cost can be considerable; in 1992, Sadler reported that a monthly prescription had cost £90. The results from the studies assessing the effectiveness of Chinese herbal medicine as a treatment for atopic eczema have shown promising results (Sheehan and Atherton, 1994). The treatment can have side effects, including potential liver damage. Many patients say that the tea is not at all pleasant to drink; some people find it so disgusting they say it is undrinkable. Some practitioners may be unregulated, and the British Association of Dermatologists has compiled a list of practitioners who are considered to be suitably qualified for assessment and treatment of patients with skin conditions. The Skin Care Campaign gives a very useful list of things to consider when deciding to approach a complementary practitioner (www.skincarecampaign.org) – for example, is the practitioner trained and qualified, and recognized by any professional body with a code of conduct?

Evening primrose oil (Epogam™) has a beneficial effect for some patients with eczema (Graham, 1984). It is now available on prescription as a treatment for atopic eczema. People with eczema tend to be less able to convert linoleic acid to gammolinoleic acid (GLA), and this can result in dry skin. Evening primrose oil is rich in essential fatty acids (namely GLA) and can therefore reduce the dry skin associated with eczema.

Mantle (1996) noted many differing treatments that patients might try. Examples included tea tree oil for acne (tea tree has antibacterial and antifungal properties), acupuncture for infantile atopic eczema, and homeopathy for psoriasis. Because people tend to feel that they are helpless to do anything about their skin, they are willing to try all sorts of different options. Some people get the desired results, while for others it is arguably a waste of time and money. So far there is little scientific research to guide the choices that people make.

Relaxation therapies

Chronic skin diseases are frequently linked to stress. A common treatment strategy throughout the years has been the amelioration of stress and the development of strategies to cope with it. This is often impractical, either because there is a problem getting the patient to identify stress or because once identified it is actually impossible to do anything about it. Historically, bed rest and sedatives accompanied by a strict topical regime was the treatment of choice for chronic skin diseases (Belk, 1983). This strategy was neither especially practical nor desirable; it did not encourage self-care, it encouraged dependence on sedatives, and it relied on the ready availability of dermatology beds for long periods of time.

Management of stress for people with skin problems has to focus on helping individuals to control or cope with stressful situations. It must be recognized that whilst the development of skin disease is often linked to stress, the presence of the visible disease is in itself a source of stress (Kirkevold, 1993). Poorman and Webb (1992) discussed how skin disease lowers self-esteem and can have a significant impact on sexuality and self-concept. Stress is an individual experience; what is stressful for one patient may not be for the next. Relaxation is a very practical way in which nurses can help patients to overcome feelings of being stressed; massage, reflexology and shiatsu are just a few of therapies through which relaxation can be attained. Introduction of relaxation therapies for patients must be done sensitively, as some will find them 'wacky' and unhelpful and may be more stressed by trying to do them than by not. Once again, it is about finding out what motivates patients and what suits their needs. In some it may be a relaxation technique, in others it may be going away on holiday.

Whatever strategy is used, it is important that patients are aware of the role that stress plays. Sometimes very practical measures, like helping them to treat their skin successfully, will reduce stress and allow resolution of the problem more quickly (Ginsburg, 1996). By learning to relax more, patients can decrease the experience of stress, which is likely to mean that their skin condition will improve. This will boost their self-confidence, encouraging them to relax further and thus show further improvement. The 'stress–skin disease–stress cycle' is a vicious circle, and nurses can play a vital role in helping to break it.

Diet

The effect of diet on the severity of eczema and other skin diseases continues to be a controversial issue. There are many anecdotal reports of the effectiveness of dietary manipulation, and it is estimated that 10–20 per cent of atopic patients *may* have some form of food allergy that acts as a trigger to their eczema (Rackett *et al.*, 1993). However, there are many people who choose dietary manipulation as an inappropriate first-line treatment for eczema. Some children are put on restrictive diets by their parents after reading unfounded claims made in newspapers and magazines. The child's development must be considered in these cases, and dietary manipulation should not be encouraged without the support of dieticians and dermatologists. There is little scientific evidence to suggest that diet has any impact on other skin conditions, although a balanced, healthy diet rich in fruit and vegetables is of course recommended.

Manipulating environmental factors

There are hazards in the home and workplace that can contribute to or exacerbate a person's skin condition, and eczema seems to be especially susceptible. However, measures can be taken to minimize the worsening of a condition by environmental factors. For example, many washing detergents, conditioners and bleaches can be irritant to a person with a skin problem. Normally people have to learn by trial and error which suits them best, but general guidelines are that non-biological powders and liquids are less irritant. Perfumed products, especially fabric condition-ers, should be avoided, and bleach tends to be particularly irritant. To reduce problems the laundry should be rinsed thor-oughly; sometimes it may be necessary to put it through an extra rinse. Hand washing can present an additional problem, since the effect of washing powders and soaps on the hands can be very irritating. Vinyl gloves (with cotton gloves inside for added protection) should be worn.

Pure cotton bed linen will help to prevent skin irritation at night. Eczema can be further exacerbated by the house dust mite, which lives in soft furnishings. People with eczema should be advised to take the following precautions, as recommended by the National Eczema Society (1994), in an attempt to diminish the harmful effects of the house dust mite:

• Air bedding and bedrooms regularly
• Use cotton blankets and sheets, and avoid the use of feather duvets and pillows because these cannot be washed
• Wash blankets at high temperatures (58°C) every 2 weeks
• Vacuum the surfaces of pillows and mattresses
• Use special mattress and duvet covers if possible, as this reduces the number of house dust mites released into the air
• Damp dust all the other surfaces in the room weekly
• Keep the number of soft toys to a minimum. Putting toys in a plastic bag and then in the freezer during the day will kill house dust mites.

Pets are a difficult issue for people with skin problems, as all furry animals can produce a reaction in patients with eczema. If the family already owns a pet and feels unable to part with it, they must be advised to restrict the movement of the animal through the house, and the sufferer's bedroom must be out of bounds. Parting with a pet may not provide an immediate solu-tion anyhow, as animal dander will exist in the house for another 2 years after the pet has gone. Families without pets should be encouraged to consider non-furry options!

When looking for clothing, patients with skin conditions should try to buy cotton because this allows a comfortable airflow and is the least irritating fabric. The person with a skin problem may have to take more time choosing clothes, carefully examining any seams, fasteners, etc. that may be rough or made of a potentially irritating substance. Jeans, for example, contain metal studs that attach buttons to the clothing, and these studs are often made of a nickel-containing metal that can irritate sensitive skin. Taking care when choosing clothing is important, as wearing comfortable fabrics will reduce the irritation of the skin.

Minimizing occupational hazards

In Northern Europe, skin problems are in the top three occupational diseases, accounting for anywhere between 9 and 34 per cent of occupational disease (Williams, 1997). The loss of days from work not only impacts on the individual and his or her family, but also on the economy. There are many skin problems caused through work, including contact dermatitis, burns and callosities (hardening of the skin through friction). Frequently these problems can be prevented by the use of protective clothing and adherence to health and safety policies.

Despite health and safety regulations and protective gear, there remain a proportion of people who will still develop occupational skin problems. Some of these can be disabling and may eventually lead to the patient stopping work. People who had atopic eczema as a child, but which has now resolved, may be at risk of developing contact dermatitis when they work in professions where they are constantly exposed to potentially irritant or sensitizing substances. Hairdressers, chefs, nurses and doctors are included in these groups. Whilst career counselling is significant for these people, it is also important that opportunities are not forsaken completely, as sometimes simple measures can be taken to reduce the risk – for example, wearing gloves when dealing with irritant substances, and using barrier creams to prevent the skin drying and cracking as well as for a degree of physical protection.

If, despite all precautionary measures, a person is being disabled by an occupational skin condition, it may be necessary to withdraw from that line of employment and consider opportunities in other fields.

Patient support groups

The large number of patient support groups available for people with skin problems reflects the amount of support that is required for coping with the conditions. Someone with a skin condition is often keen to substantiate the advice given by the GP or other healthcare professional. Directing patients to a recognized body of information means that they are more likely to receive good advice rather than relying on the often erroneous suggestions made by television, magazines and friends. NHS Direct offers a number of services, including telephone information (tele-phone 0845 46 47) and an online service (www.nhsdirect.nhs.uk). Both services continue to develop, and provide an excellent and accessible source of information.

There are support groups for the majority of skin problems, including psoriasis, eczema, vitiligo and acne. The groups pro-vide literature for patients, there is often a newsletter, and some have local support networks that arrange meetings and raise money. Research often relies on the money raised locally for fund-ing. In recognition of the need for increased education amongst staff the National Eczema Society has commenced training days for nurses, with speakers from the healthcare professions and patient groups (Contact the National Eczema Society for further details). Names and addresses of support groups are given in Appendix A.

The specific groups aim to support patients with specific conditions, but the Skin Care Campaign has a more general approach, concerning itself with assuring the highest possible standards of healthcare provision for people with skin disease (Skin Care Campaign website, www.skincarecampaign.org). This is done by working with patient and professional organ-izations, and with the pharmaceutical industry. Campaigning is carried out through a number of channels, including the Associate Parliamentary Group on Skin (formerly the All Party Parliamentary Group on Skin); educate and inform through the media; and encourage the provision of more information for patients through their Skin Information Days.

Financial assistance

The treatment of skin problems usually involves more that one item on prescription. A patient may have to spend over £50 after one consultation. Whilst it may seem excessive, it is not unusual for a patient of be prescribed a bath emollient, soap substitute, moisturizer, two strengths of topical steroid, a scalp treatment, shampoo, antihistamines and antibiotics. This would be a basic set of treatments; the patient may find that they do not work or run out quickly, and will then have to return to the clinic within a few weeks to be prescribed further treatments.

The cost can soon mount up, and this can be a very serious problem for someone with a low disposable income. Many patients have to make difficult choices between paying for their prescrip-tion or for other necessities such as food or bills. Unsurprisingly, many people do without the prescription. Patients with skin conditions are not entitled to free prescriptions, unlike many other people with chronic conditions such as epilepsy and diabetes. This puts an added burden onto someone who is already likely to be stressed by a disfiguring condition.

Patients should be advised that some items can be purchased over the counter at a lower cost than the prescription charge. There are a range of moisturizers (e.g. '50/50' – 50% per cent white soft paraffin, 50 per cent liquid paraffin and aqueous cream) that are cheaper to purchase this way, but there are a number that are actually more expensive than the prescription charge (e.g. E45 and Cetreban™), especially if purchasing the larger-sized containers. Patients should be encouraged to check that they are not exempt from paying prescription charges; it is a good idea to ask their GP or visit the Citizens' Advice Bureau. It is also possible to get a pre-payment certificate, which means paying up front for prescriptions; in general, if patients have more than five items on prescription in 3 months it is a cheaper way to get prescription items. Forms can be obtained from the local health authority, and some pharmacists may stock them.

Cosmetic assistance for patients with alopecia (baldness) or vitiligo (loss of skin pigment) is crucial in many people's lives. The application of make-up or the wearing of a wig hides disfigurement, allowing the patient to avoid constant staring from the inquisitive public. Patients can obtain some assistance in the purchase of these products. The camouflage make-up is available on prescription, and there are clinics in some NHS Trusts that teach patients how to apply it; the British Red Cross also provides a voluntary service. Wigs can be prescribed through the NHS when the patient suffers from alopecia totalis or alopecia areata (sudden hair loss). A wig can be prescribed through the hospital's wig agency, but many patients find that they are not happy with the quality of NHS wigs. Some Trusts offer a voucher scheme, where patients can choose any wig and pay the difference in price between this and the NHS allowance. It is important for patients' morale that they find a wig that they are happy with so that they can wear it with confidence.

There are a number of benefits available if a skin problem causes severe difficulties for the person in the home. A person with a chronic skin problem may have difficulties at work, with increased time off due to sickness, or, more seriously, be totally unable to work. Often skin conditions mean that more money has to be spent on bed linen and clothes, which are ruined by treatments. The washing machine and vacuum cleaner are in constant use and therefore will need replacing and/or fixing sooner, and all-cotton clothing is often more expensive than synthetic fabrics. It is not hard to see how someone with a skin condition can find themselves in serious financial difficulties.

Government assistance comes in the form of the Disability Living Allowance, which is not means-tested and may be awarded to people who need to be cared for. Invalid Care Allowance is paid to a carer if he or she spends more than 35 hours a week caring for someone. The DSS has a free telephone enquiry number through which patients can discuss their needs (0800 88 22 00), and a leaflet (N1196) covers all the Social Security benefit rates. Independent organizations may be of some help in awarding grants in exceptional circumstances. Families with a child who is severely affected by atopic eczema or epidermolysis bullosa sometimes qualify for these allowances and grants.

There is therefore very little statutory financial help for those with skin problems, despite the extra expense that it can incur. Stress is linked with skin problems, a further difficulties of financing treatment must be a further burden to many patients, potentially exacerbating their condition even more.

Conclusion

This chapter has examined the many challenges that patients face when they attempt to treat their skin at home. Changes in health-care provision over the past few years have seen a reduction in dermatology beds and therefore an increase in the number of patients juggling their topical treatments with their daily routines. The treatments tend to be complex and messy, requiring a strong and motivated individual to be able to continue applica-tion everyday. The support of the patient's family and of health-care professionals is important in achieving successful patient concordance. The patient is also faced with the media, who encourage the questioning of prescribed medications and offer dubious cures to vulnerable people. There are complementary therapies that are having some success in providing relief for people with certain skin conditions, for example Chinese herbal medicine. However, the mainstay of treatment remains the daily application of topical treatments. This can be made much easier if nurses helping the patients are knowledgeable and sympathetic about their skin problems.

Reflective activities

1. Consider the implications on the home life of a young couple who have a child diagnosed with atopic eczema. How would you explain the condition and treatments to the couple? What other help may be available?
2. Imagine you are a teenager who is attending the GP's surgery because of some scaly red patches that have appeared on your face and body. What do you (as the teenager) feel are the most important issues that the consultation should focus on?
3. You are a district nurse visiting an elderly patient who has just attended a dermatology clinic and has been prescribed a bath oil, soap substitute, two moisturizers (one for day and one for night), two topical steroids for 1 week, and a new regime for the following week. How would you ensure that the patient was able to follow the regime, and what sort of support would you offer?
4. Think how a patient may feel when prescribed a new treatment. The label warns that it may stain clothing and it has a very strong smell when the lid is removed. This patient has to wear a smart suit to work and, although motivated to do the treatments, is concerned about the smell and how people might react to this. How do you think the patient can overcome these problems and treat the skin complaint?

References

All Party Parliamentary Group on Skin. (1998). *Enquiry into the Training of Health Care Professionals Who Come into Contact with Skin Diseases*. APPG.

Belk, D. (1983). Nursing care study: psoriasis. *Nursing Times*, **79(10)**, 49–53.

Bowman, J. (1994). More than skin deep. *Nursing Times*, **90(23)**, 43–6.

British Association of Dermatologists. (1994). *Report of the BAD London Dermatology Services Working Party*. BAD.

British National Formulary. (1998) No. 32. British Medical Association and Royal Pharmaceutical Society of Great Britain.

Davis, H. and Fallowfield, L. (1991). *Counselling and Communication in Health Care*. John Wiley and Sons.

Department of Health. (1999). *Saving Lives: Our Healthier Nation*. HMSO.

Department of Health. (2000). *The NHS Plan – A Plan for Investment, A Plan for Reform*. The Stationery Office Ltd.

Dermatological Care Working Group. (2001). *Assessment of Best Practice for Dermatology Services in Primary Care*. Ash Associates.

Frost, J. (1994). Complementary treatments for eczema in children. *Prof. Nurse*, **9(5)**, 330–32.

Gawkrodger, D. J. (1992). *An Illustrated Colour Text: Dermatology*. Churchill Livingstone.

Ginsburg, I. H. (1996). The psychosocial impact of skin disease: an overview. *Dermatol. Clin.*, **14(3)**, 473–84.

Graham, J. (1984). *Eczema* Thornson's, London.

Jowett, S. and Ryan, T. (1985). Skin disease and handicap. *Soc. Sci. Med.*, **20(4)**, 425–9.

Kirkevold, M. (1993). Toward a practice theory of caring for patient with chronic skin disease. *Scholarly inquiry for Nursing Practice*, **7(1)**, 37–52.

Laffrey, S. C., Bailey, B. J. and Craig, K. K. (1996). Social support and health promotion: outcomes of adults with psoriasis. *Dermatol. Nursing*, **8(2)**, 109–12, 117–119, 143.

Lawton, S. (1999). How to ... wet wrap. *Br. J. Dermatol. Nursing*, **3(1)**, 8–9.

Long, C. C. and Finlay, A. Y. (1992). The fingertip unit: a new practical measure. *Clin. Exper. Dermatol.*, **16(6)**, 444–7.

Mantle, F. (1996). More than skin deep. *Nursing Times*, **92(36)**, 56–7.

Mitchell, T., Paige, D. and Spowart, K. (1998). *Eczema and your Child*. Class Publishing.

National Eczema Society. (1994). *The Management and Treatment of Eczema*. National Eczema Society.

Niven, N. (1989). *Health Psychology: An Introduction for Nurses and Other Health Care Professionals*. Churchill Livingstone.

Penzer, R. (2000). Improving quality of care in chronic skin conditions. *Nursing Standard*. **15(12)**, 33.

Poorman, S. G. and Webb, C. A. (1992). Sexuality and self concept: issues in skin disease. *Dermatol. Nursing*, **4(4)**, 279–84.

Rackett, S. C., Rothe, M. J. and Grant-Kels, J. M. (1993). Diet and dermatology. *J. Am. Acad. Dermatol.*, **29(3)**, 447–61.

Royal College of General Practitioners. (1995). *Morbidity Statistics from General Practice: Fourth National Study 1991–92*. HMSO.

Ruane-Morris, M. (1995). Nurses' perceptions of dermatology. *Prof. Nurse*, **10(8)**, 501–4.

Sackett, D. L. and Snow, J. C. (1989). The magnitude of compliance and non-compliance. In Haynes, R. B., Taylor, D. W., Sackett, D., eds. *Compliance in Healthcare*, Johns Hopkins University Press, Baltimore.

Sadler, C. (1992). Time for tea? *Nursing Times*, **85(35)**, 34–6.

Sheehan, M. P. and Atherton, D. (1994). One year follow-up of children treated with Chinese medicinal herbs for atopic eczema. *Br. J. Dermatol.*, **130(4)**, 488–93.

van Onselen, J. (1998). Working towards patient concordance. *Br. J. Dermatol. Nursing*, **2(1)**, 2.

Venables, J. (1995). The management and treatment of eczema. *Nursing Standard*, **9(4)**, 25–8.

Williams, H. C. (1997). *Dermatology: Health Care Needs Assessment*. Radcliffe Medical Press.

Wright, A. (1992). *Topical Steroids Exchange*, **67**, 8–9. National Eczema Society.

Websites

Royal Pharmaceutical Society. (2000) www.concordance.org

Skin Care Campaign. (2000). www.skincarecampaign.org

Health promotion in skin care

Pauline Buchanan

Introduction

Nursing in the 1990s brought about many developments and changes. Arguably the most important development is the change in emphasis from nursing ill health to promoting positive health.

(Macleod-Clark, 1993)

Health promotion now features strongly in all areas of clinical practice. Traditionally, health visitors, occupational health nurses and primary care nurses have been seen to adopt a health promotion role. Clearly, however, it is now recognized that there is a role for health promotion for all nurses regardless of clinical specialty. Indeed, the long-term, relapsing nature of many chronic skin conditions demands that health professionals direct interventions towards care and prevention rather than cure. That in itself promotes a vital health promotion role. Therefore, the main aim in providing nursing care is to assist patients and families to cope with, adapt or adjust to their skin condition.

This chapter aims to clarify the key nursing roles in health promotion, and review the strategies available to nurses, through discussion of theories of health promotion. In relating these theories to specific areas of practice, the role of the nurse in health promotion will be clearly identified.

Approaches to health promotion

Several theories of health promotion are now recognized and offer model approaches to care (French and Adams, 1986). Those most frequently cited are the medical, behavioural, educational and social change models. All these models aim to bring about behavioural change leading to healthier living. Although relating these theories to clinical practice is often complex, these models are worthy of further discussion as they provide a framework for care and evaluation which is important in nursing today.

Medical approach

Becker describes one behavioural approach in his health belief model (Becker, 1974), which offers the theory that we are motivated to avoid ill health for fear of the consequences. This model focuses on disease, and aims to reduce mortality and morbidity associated with disease or illness. The health belief model promotes healthier lifestyles through changes in behaviour, which are based on perceived susceptibility, severity and benefits, and the costs of modifying a behaviour. Individuals weigh up the benefits of changing their behaviour to a healthier lifestyle against the risks or costs of no change. If they perceive the risks of disease, illness or injury as being greater than the benefits of their existing lifestyle, then a change in behaviour is likely. For example, patients with psoriasis who have extremely stressful lifestyles frequently report that stress acts as a 'trigger' to relapse. The benefits and costs of reducing the stress within their life have to be weighed up against the likelihood of continued stress adversely affecting the psoriasis. This can be difficult as other influencing factors are involved, such as family/friends, financial considerations, personality and self-concept.

The health belief model favours a medical approach to intervention in health promotion, with screening/immunization programmes and presentation of facts, figures and statistics, and fails to recognize influencing social factors. Health education messages may be negative in nature, which is one criticism of this model; therefore many health promotion workers favour behavioural, educational and/or social approaches.

Behavioural approach

The main aim of a behavioural approach is to change people's attitudes and behaviour and thus guide them towards better health and/or lifestyles (Ewles and Simnet, 1985). This can be achieved through the acquisition of knowledge and information. A behavioural approach recognizes the influence of beliefs, attitudes and significant others on existing behaviours and/or intended behaviours. There are several models related to behavioural approaches, and these are described in this section.

The theory of reasoned action model (Ajzen and Fishbein, 1980) supports this approach and values the influence of others in promoting behaviour change. This is an interesting point from a nursing perspective in that group work, patient peer support and mutual support groups (self-help) are commonplace in health care. Such approaches to care serve to increase knowledge and understanding, promote psychosocial support and increase individual self-esteem.

Poor self-concept (self-esteem and body image) can be evident in persons with chronic skin conditions. The importance of high self-esteem in facilitating behaviour change is emphasized in the health action model (Tones, 1987); the lower the self-esteem, the less motivated the individual is to change behaviour or even take notice of the health education message. This can frequently become an important nursing issue when caring for someone with skin problems, as self-concept is very often diminished. Nursing interventions are aimed at positively influencing the patient's self-esteem and body image, which in turn may motivate the patient to adopt more appropriate behaviours.

Prochaska and DiClemente (1984) describe the different stages individuals pass through when intending to change behaviour – pre-contemplation, contemplation, action, maintenance and relapse. These stages relate to a person's thought (cognitive) processes, attitude, belief and eventual behaviour changes. The pre-contemplation stage is seen as the phase when a person is not seriously considering a change in behaviour or is unaware that a behaviour change is necessary. Contemplation occurs when a person demonstrates awareness of a problem requiring a behaviour change, but is not as yet fully committed to the action. In the action stage, which follows contemplation, overt behaviour change is apparent. Maintenance represents a continuance of the behaviour change, and relapse occurs if and when maintenance behaviours fail. The length of time a person remains in each phase or stage is individual and varies, and therefore the main aim of the nurse as health promoter is to empower patients or individuals to identify the stage reached and facilitate further change when needed. This self-awareness can threate an individual's self-esteem, especially during the contemplation and relapse phases. However, successful action and maintenance behaviours positively influence self-esteem, thus promoting health.

Educational approach

Thompson (1983) supports the concept of an educational approach in health promotion, as it attempts to be value-free so that an informed choice can be made by the individual and then acted upon. Clearly the medical, educational and behavioural approaches are not mutually exclusive, as they all require an educational component. Knowledge and understanding facilitates behaviour change. The enormous mushrooming in availability and diversity of patient information leaflets, posters and literature is evidence of an educational approach to health promotion.

Social change approach

This approach identifies policy makers as agents of change. These policy makers may be targeted within the family, communities or at government level. Strategies focus on environmental issues, policies and widespread multimedia campaigns. The Australian national sun awareness/skin cancer prevention campaigns of the last few years are ongoing and aim to change undesirable behaviours (overexposure to sunshine) through a social change approach – e.g. a 'no hat no play' policy in schools. However, there are also behavioural, educational and medical components to these campaigns, and this clearly illustrates the value of an eclectic approach to health promotion.

The nurse's role in health promotion

It may be useful to identify clinical areas where nurses can perform the health promotion role with regard to skin conditions and disease. Dermatology as a clinical speciality within secondary healthcare services is seen as a unique and highly specialized area of practice. Clinical nurse specialists in dermatology are few, as are dermatology wards. Changing times, resources, and the nature of chronic skin conditions have seen a shift from inpatient care to outpatient management, which may incorporate hospital-based daily treatments. Ninety-five per cent of all dermatology cases are managed on an outpatient basis. Therefore nurses involved in managing these patients may be involved in other clinical specialties such as medical or paediatric nursing, outpatients' departments, primary care and occupational health. Many Trusts provide or allocate 'dermatology beds' within acute care or rehabilitation wards. Therefore is important that all nurses, and not only those specializing in dermatology, have a good understanding of health promotion issues when caring for patients with skin conditions. It should also be recognized that all nurses have a role in health promotion regarding skin care, even in the absence of overt skin disease.

Disease prevention

The concept of disease prevention, the alternative view of health promotion, is traditionally classified into three main groups, primary, secondary and tertiary, and relates to the preventive strategies utilized and the disease stage (Muir-Gray and Fowler, 1984).

Primary prevention of disease

Primary prevention of disease aims to prevent disease occurring altogether, and therefore the target population consists of healthy individuals. Examples of primary prevention are the immunization programmes for rubella and measles, two of the most common childhood skin diseases. This form of disease prevention focuses on the acute infectious skin diseases (bacterial and viral), some of which have been eradicated from Britain due to successful immunization and education campaigns (e.g. smallpox). Primary prevention occurs, to a large extent, in primary care.

The single most important primary preventive strategy is health education, and this underpins all health promotion. Health education is discussed in detail later in this chapter.

Secondary prevention of disease

The health promotion strategies employed here are specifically targeted towards the diagnosis of early disease and the implementation of appropriate treatments. Clearly, secondary preventive strategies represent a major focus for nurses in identifying early skin disease or problems. Whether in acute care, primary health care or occupational health, the early identification of skin problems is a nursing responsibility.

Breakdown of skin integrity is frequently cited as a potential nursing problem due to recumbence, associated disease, trauma or age. Nursing assessments of skin integrity and associated risk factors are good examples of secondary prevention, and are recognized in clinical practice with the widespread implementation of a variety of assessment scales such as Norton's assessment tool (Norton *et al.*, 1975).

Nursing assessments regarding skin integrity are vital in the early diagnosis of a variety of dermatological conditions. For example, infestations (e.g. lice and scabies) and infections (fungal, viral or bacterial) may be suspected by the attending nurse, who then promptly initiates referral to a medical practitioner for diagnosis and treatment. Similarly, the early recognition and intervention for skin conditions such as psoriasis and eczema may well reduce the psychosocial morbidity associated with these chronic diseases.

Delay in diagnosis is an important issue in skin care. Many skin conditions have an insidious onset, and are initially symptom-free and non-life threatening. This leads to delay in seeking medical advice and eventual chronicity of disease (e.g. tinea pedis developing from athlete's foot) and more complex and longer-term management (e.g. in psoriasis and eczema). More alarmingly, delay in diagnosis of skin cancer, especially malignant melanoma, can lead to disfigurement and fewer treatment options, and can be potentially life threatening. The Government's White Paper *Health of the Nation* identified skin cancer as a serious health problem in the white adult population (Department of Health, 1992). The *Health of the Nation* target for skin cancer is to 'to reduce the year on year increase in incidence by the year 2005'. Since its publication, widespread local and national public education campaigns have been initiated in order to facilitate early diagnosis and treatment of malignant melanoma.

Tertiary prevention of disease

This represents the traditional nursing role in the care and management of patients with overt disease. Preventive strategies are aimed at reducing further deterioration, preventing complications and improving health. Nursing care is holistic in nature, and addresses the physical, emotional, psychological and spiritual needs of the patients in order to prevent psychological morbidity such as anxiety, depression and resentment.

Health promotion roles in nursing

The health promotion role of all nurses involved in caring for patients' skin consists of a variety of sub-roles, all of which are important. However, more emphasis may be placed on certain sub-roles as is demanded by the individual situation.

These sub-roles for health promotion can be categorized as direct or indirect patient care.

Direct patient care

Nursing a patient with skin problems demands that the nurse be a competent clinical practitioner, incorporating holistic care for patients and their families. Emotional support for patients and their families is integral to care, as fears and anxieties may trigger or exacerbate the skin condition. Therefore time, patience and an understanding of their fears and concerns are essential. Only then can individual coping mechanisms be identified in order to help the patient develop a positive outlook. Talking to the patient and family, sensitively touching the patient's skin and dispelling any myths such as cross-infection, if appropriate, are all very important. Isolation in a single room because of skin disease is not always appropriate, and indeed may fuel fears and anxieties about being contagious.

Regular contact with patients both on an individual basis and in group sessions will incorporate the sub-roles of nursing adviser, patient's advocate and health educator. The most important of these is health educator, as health education is integral to all nursing and features strongly in primary, secondary and tertiary disease prevention programmes.

Health education

The relationship between health education and health promotion is not always clear, although health education can be defined as the essential communicational component of any preventive medicine (Anderson, 1979). This concept is supported by the generally accepted view that health education serves to promote an understanding of health and aims to modify individuals' behaviour, which will help to prevent disease. Health education is therefore only one component of health promotion, but represents the cornerstone of all other health promotion strategies (Maben and Macleod-Clark, 1995).

The main objectives of health education in skin care are:

1. To increase patients' knowledge and understanding of their skin condition and its management
2. To facilitate early diagnosis of potential problems/complications
3. To commence treatment and care promptly in order to prevent deterioration, promote healing and increase the length of remission periods
4. To modify patients' behaviours in order to promote future health.

Ultimately, the main aim of all health education is to reduce physical and psychological morbidity associated with the disease or condition.

One area where health education has been deemed successful is skin cancer prevention. A Californian study (Temoshok *et al.*, 1984) highlighted certain factors associated with patient delay in seeking medical advice regarding malignant melanoma. First, patients with no (or limited) knowledge of malignant melanoma, had significantly thicker lesions at presentation than patients with some knowledge. Secondly, patients with less understanding of its treatment had significantly thicker lesions and delayed longer before seeking medical advice. Finally, and very interestingly, patients who downplayed the seriousness of their disease delayed less. A possible explanation of this is that minimizing the seriousness of the condition reduces anxiety and fears, thus making the idea of treatment less frightening. Similarly, within the UK a Glasgow study (Docherty and Mackie, 1986) attributed poor prognosis of malignant melanoma to patient delay, and, following an intensive education campaign, a significantly greater number of thinner 'good' prognosis lesions were diagnosed. One explanation for this finding is that the informed population developed a greater understanding of melanoma, treatments and prognosis, and therefore sought medical advice promptly.

A Skin Cancer Prevention Working Party is now established in the UK, and Health Commissions throughout the country have nominated skin cancer prevention officers whose main remit is to direct local public and professional education programmes. Clearly this represents a vital area where health education can prevent disease, and should be addressed by every nurse within the profession. Results from the ongoing research and prevention campaigns in response to *Health of the Nation* have yet to be published, but it is hoped that the incidence and mortality rates of malignant melanoma will be significantly reduced. Such changes can be achieved through the behaviour modification highlighted in all educational campaigns. The current Health Education Authority 'Sun know-how' campaign is a good example of how health education focuses on behaviour change to prevent disease (Health Education Authority, 1996). The key message in this campaign is to 'shift to the shade' by avoiding sunburn and midday sun exposure, and wearing wide-brimmed hats, tee-shirts, sunglasses and sunscreens.

Chronic skin conditions

Although skin cancer prevention represents an excellent example of the importance of nurses' health education role, the same principles apply to all areas of nursing. Increasing patient knowledge and understanding in the management of chronic skin conditions such as psoriasis and eczema will lead to greater patient compliance, greater efficacy of treatments and greater patient satisfaction. A prerequisite to the above is identifying the patient's needs, whether educational, physical or emotional.

As mentioned previously, the skin and the psyche are closely linked, and stress, anxieties or fears can worsen skin conditions. These fears and anxieties may be alleviated or reduced if caused by knowledge deficit. Specific stressors that exacerbate the condition can be identified, and coping mechanisms recognized, as part of a stress management programme. Education and support on stress management may empower patients to examine aspects of their life (career, financial, relationships, self-concept) that contribute to overall stress. The chronicity of disease makes stress management and psychosocial support a major nursing consideration, as no cure can be offered for genetically determined conditions (e.g. psoriasis and atopic eczema). Learning to live with the chronic skin condition represents the greatest challenge for all patients.

There is a wider challenge here for nurses using health education for those with chronic skin disease. Providing health education is not just about changing behaviour but also about empowering patients to use knowledge to alter their experience of ill health. For example, if patients are taught how to apply moisturizers so that their skin is less dry, flaky and unsightly, they may feel more accepted by society and less isolated. The improved sense of well-being could in turn decrease their stress levels and further enhance their ability to partake in their own care, thus improving the outcome of the physical treatments. This may then lead to an increased sense of well-being and decrease in stress. A positive cycle of events is set up, allowing patients a better quality of life.

It can be seen that greater understanding of the disease and its management, and reducing exposure to trigger factors, are the long-term nurse and patient goals. The desired outcome is to ameliorate some of the psychosocial problems associated with chronic skin conditions, such as anxiety, frustration, anger and depression. These feelings, which are expressions of emotional stress, can further exacerbate the skin condition. This emotional stress can be felt by other family members, who may experience feelings of guilt, hostility and rejection, and family relationships can be affected and feelings of hopelessness become evident. Addressing emotional stress is a vital part of management for patients and families. If these problems can be avoided, patients' self-esteem and body image will be positively affected, with greater social recovery, a return to work, and improved satisfaction with their life.

Cultural considerations

A further consideration in promoting health relates to culture. Recognition and acceptance of cultural influences on individuals, their skin disease and their way of life will enhance the success of health education or another health promotion strategy. Culture is a term that incorporates numerous concepts such as behaviours, beliefs, attitudes, language, values, religion, socialization, diet, ideologies, rituals, rules, institutions, education, art, literature and artefacts (Chandler, 1991). Working within a multicultural society, nurses, as health promoters, should be aware of the differences and similarities in cultures. It is a nursing responsibility to identify:

- Specific cultural values in relation to health promotion
- Susceptibility to skin disease
- Health and illness beliefs and practices.

Nursing interventions that focus on these issues of health promotion aim to improve the quality of life for patients and their families.

Indirect patient care

Health promotion nursing sub-roles in this category include acting as a change agent, supervisor, clinical teacher, researcher, liaison officer, innovator and resource person. These sub-roles are not mutually exclusive, and the role of liaison officer can be considered the most important because it incorporates all other roles to some degree, the main objective being to disseminate knowledge and nursing skills to colleagues, patients and their families.

Chronic skin conditions require long-term medical follow-up, multidisciplinary approaches to care, and ongoing nursing support. Therefore it is important to ensure that adequate support, reassurance and information is provided for patients and fellow professionals. One method of facilitating this is to provide written information leaflets that outline the nature of the disease and the importance of treatments, and give information regarding where help and advice can be sought (e.g. self-help groups, local nurse specialists and national charities). However, written information is not considered a replacement for the spoken word, and should act as a reinforcement to all direct nursing interventions.

Summary of nursing responsibilities

In summary, the main nursing responsibilities for health promotion when nursing patients with skin problems are as follows:

1. Assess the patient's individual physical, psychological, emotional and spiritual needs

2. Plan health promotion strategies according to the patient's identified needs
3. Implement appropriate primary, secondary and tertiary preventive strategies
4. Evaluate health promotion nursing interventions in behavioural terms: patient compliance, level of knowledge and understanding.

A model way forward

Nursing a patient with skin disease demands that the whole person is cared for, and not just the skin condition. Therefore, the physical, psychological, emotional and spiritual aspects of care need to be addressed. This can be achieved through application of the nursing process and the use of a model of nursing. A systematic approach to care is recommended in all nursing settings. Health promotion can be incorporated into care plans by applying a nursing theory. Theory-based practice is recommended, as it will establish clinical competence and allow the nurse to use independent judgement, be reflective in practice, and maintain credibility.

One of the most popular theories used in nursing is Roper's activities of daily living (Roper *et al.*, 1990). Ease of application to clinical settings is this model's main advantage. It is simple to understand and implement; however it may be criticized in that it focuses on the physical aspects of care, with little emphasis being placed on the psychological or emotional aspects. Roy's adaptation model (Roy, 1984), Neuman's systems model (Neuman, 1989) or Orem's self-care model (Orem, 1985) may be more appropriate when caring for someone with skin disease.

A theoretical framework for health promotion must also to be considered if health education is to be incorporated into care planning. As previously discussed, one drawback of Becker's health belief model is that it is medical in nature and focuses on disease. The more positive aspects of health can be lost by negative and threatening health education messages.

An educational/behavioural approach or model may be more appropriate in dermatology, as it promotes the affective and cognitive aspects of learning in health education. In utilizing this approach nurses can recognize and acknowledge patients' beliefs, values and feelings, which aid individual learning and behaviour modification. Orem's self-care model represents a good example of how this may be achieved.

Orem's model applied to skin care

The use of a model of nursing demands in-depth analysis of individualized care. Although it would be possible to use a number of models, Orem's self-care model is very appropriate for health promotion, as the self-care philosophy offers direction for improved health within individuals and families (Denyes, 1988).

The strengths of Orem's model for use as a health promotion tool relate to delivery of care. Three categories of nursing intervention are identified: fully compensatory, partially compensatory, and supportive/educative care.

Fully compensatory care is recognized as the care provided by someone other than the patient, known as the self-care agent, such as nurse, parent or carer. The patient's responsibility to self-care is temporarily relieved, and the self-care agent meets all health needs – for example when a patient is acutely ill, or when caring for a young child.

As a patient's self-care abilities increase, the care provided by the nurse or carer is described as partially compensatory. Gradually, full self-care responsibilities will be undertaken by the individual patient. Implicit to fully compensatory and partially compensatory care is the supportive and educative mode of nursing, where the nurse or carer meets the psychosocial needs of the patient. Even if a patient does not need physical care, nursing help with learning deficits may still be necessary through educational support. Thus the supportive/educative role can take place when the patient is fully self-caring otherwise, or as part of the fully or partly compensatory stages.

The Orem philosophy of care lends itself well to nursing, where different levels of intervention are required depending on the patient's self-care ability. Throughout, the supportive-educative aspects of care emphasize the importance of health education. The following example (Tables 6.1, 6.2) aims to provide a clear illustration of holistic care for a patient with acute exacerbation of eczema, incorporating an individual/family-centred approach and addressing issues such as stress management through an educational/behavioural approach.

The example represents a core care plan and can be adapted for use in any clinical setting. The care plan clearly identifies assessment, planning, implementation and evaluation of care, essential components of the nursing process. The modes of nursing intervention clarifies and operationalizes Orem's theory of nursing which incorporates the importance of health promotion by utilizing an educational, behavioural and social approach to change.

Conclusion

This chapter has dealt mainly with the role of the nurse in health promotion, with the principal focus being the management of patients with skin problems. Health education has been highlighted as the single most important component of health promotion, and is integral to all primary, secondary and tertiary preventive strategies. The nature of chronic skin diseases demands a holistic approach to care, as skin disease affects every aspect of the patient's life, including their psyche. Health promotion is integral to all nursing interventions, yet is frequently given little emphasis. The specific psychosocial problems experienced by patients with skin problems can be resolved or reduced if the nurse demonstrates understanding and awareness of their patients' emotional and psychological needs. The application of the nursing process and/or nursing model gives direction to the health promotion provided within care. There is no doubt that there is a place for health promotion when caring for patients with chronic skin conditions and in the prevention of skin malignancies.

Reflective activities

1. Review the nursing care plan in this chapter, and identify which nursing interventions can be classified as primary, secondary or tertiary prevention of disease.
2. Review the nursing care plan for a patient/client with a skin disease/condition under your care:

   • Identify the patient problems and categorize identified needs as physical, psychological, emotional or spiritual
   • Consider whether any nursing intervention involves health promotion for skin care
   • Identify the health promotion strategies you would use to prevent further skin problems (e.g. assessment tools, education, screening).

3. Review the skin care policies for patients and staff within your working environment:

   • Identify any problems associated with existing policies
   • What health promotion measures may be implemented to further improve skin care for patients and staff?
   • Discuss your ideas, thoughts or plans with your colleagues and clinical manager.

Table 6.1 Orem nursing assessment and planning (Orem, 1985)

Orem nursing assessment and planning: Patient name   Hospital no.   Date

Self-care demand	Self-care ability	Self-care deficit		Predicted self-care ability
Universal requisites	Initial assessment	Actual problem/need	Potential problem/need	Expected outcome/goal
Air	Full self-care ability	Nil		Prevent further deterioration in skin condition/infection; promote healing; reduce pruritus and inflammation; restore normal activity sleep pattern
Water	Full self-care ability	Nil		
Food	Full self-care ability	Nil		
Elimination	Full self-care ability	Nil		
Activity and rest	Inability to obtain adequate sleep, disruption in activity rest balance	Skin condition, pruritus and discomfort disrupting sleep pattern, causing tiredness and fatigue	Long-term sleep deprivation increases anxiety, reduces ability to avoid excoriation of skin, increases potential for infection	
Solitude and social	Disruption in social interactions	Anxiety/depression due to skin condition and pruritus affecting self-concept and social interactions causing feelings of embarrassment. Increased periods of isolation	Long-term anxiety, solitude, poor self-concept, potential risk of depression, feelings of anger, guilt and helplessness	Reduce anxiety; increase patient knowledge and understanding of skin condition and management; facilitate expression of feelings and thoughts

Hazards to well-being	Deterioration in skin condition represents a hazard to well-being and human functioning	Breakdown in skin integrity, inflammation, pruritus and anxiety are hazards to well-being and human functioning	Patient is at risk of widespread skin infection due to breakdown in skin integrity	Reduction in inflammation, pruritus and discomfort; no expression or evidence of stress or anxiety; no evidence of excoriated/infected skin.
Development, potential normality	Breakdown in skin integrity adversely affecting human normality/development and potential	Acute feelings of loss of control in self care during active phases of skin condition; chronic nature of skin condition adversely affecting self-concept, social activities and human potential	Potential long-term risk of poor self image and self-esteem, which will affect human functioning and development within social groups and personal relationships	Expression and utilization of normal coping mechanisms; normal functioning within social groups; no expression of dissatisfaction with self-concept or personal relationships

Table 6.2 Nursing care

Self-care deficit / Patient problem/need	Nurse/patient goal	Nursing interventions — Wholly compensatory	Nursing interventions — Partial compensatory	Nursing interventions — Supportive/educative	Evaluation and review date
1. Breakdown in skin integrity = hazard to human well-being and functioning	1. Prevent further deterioration and promote healing in skin condition	1. Apply moisturizers and topical medications to affected areas as prescribed; apply tubular gauze bandages to limbs and trunk	1. Explain and demonstrate application of moisturizers and topical medications in preparation for self care/home care following acute stage	1. Teach patient and carers differences between care of dry skin and eczema; outline rational for moisturization, treatment creams and bandaging	1. Reduction in extent of erythema scaling, excoriation; reduction in dry skin; no evidence of infection. Review: 24 hours
2. Pruritus = hazard to human well-being and human functioning. Alterations in activity and rest balance	2. Reduce pruritus and break scratch–cycle; promote balance between rest and activity	2. Ensure emollient bath and soap substitute is incorporated into moisturization regimen; introduce non-invasive techniques to control pruritus; administer antihistamine medication as prescribed	2. Encourage moisturization programme as daily routine before and after discharge from hospital; practise non-invasive techniques to control pruritus with patient	2. Clarify anti-pruritic, anti-inflammatory effect of moisturization and topical steroids; encourage patient and carers to employ distraction therapies and relaxation techniques	2. Reduction in pruritus and excoriation; patient using 'pat' technique; patient and carers using distraction therapies. Review: 24 hours

3. Anxiety = hazard to human well-being and human functioning	3. Alleviate anxiety	3. Ensure adequate sleep and rest during acute stage; incorporate rest periods into daily regimen; administer medication as prescribed	3. Discuss normal coping mechanisms for patient and carers; demonstrate and practise relaxation techniques for carers and patient; identify areas of knowledge deficit	3. Encourage patient to employ relaxed approach to care; outline strategies to ensure skin is not focus of attention; educate patient in areas of knowledge deficit	3. Patient and carers show a clear understanding of skin care, pruritus and eczema; no sign of stress or anxiety associated with skin state. Review: 48 hours
4. Breakdown in skin integrity = detrimental effect on human functioning and development within social groups, human potential and desire for normality	4. Promote personal development and social functioning	4. Identify social situations and activities patient and family enjoy; identify social situations in which patient feels uncomfortable or unable to participate	4. Discuss social situations and activities with patient; discuss coping strategies	4. Identify and discuss strategies that will facilitate increased social functioning at home/work/school/college/leisure	4. Patient and carers able to develop social interactions and resume activities previously ceased. Review: 7–14 days

References

Ajzen, I. and Fishbein, M. (1980). *Understanding Attitudes and Predicting Social Behaviour*. Prentice Hall.

Anderson, D. C. (1979). Chapter 1. In: *Health Education in Practice* (D. C. Anderson, ed.), p. 13. Croom Helm.

Becker, M. H. (1974). The health belief model and sick role behaviour. *Health Education Monographs*, **Winter**, 411–19.

Chandler, J. (1991). *Tabbner's Nursing Care: Theory and Practice*, pp. 61–63. Churchill Livingstone.

Denyes, M. J. (1988). Orem's model used for health promotion: directions from research. *Adv. Nursing Sci.*, **11(1)**, 13–21.

Department of Health (1992). *Health of the Nation: A Strategy for Health* in England. HMSO.

Docherty, V. R. and Mackie, R. M. (1986). Reasons for poor prognosis in British patients with cutaneous malignant melanoma. *Br. J. Med.*, **292**, 987–9.

Ewles, L. and Simnett, J. (1985). *Promoting Health: A Practical Guide to Health Education*, pp. 30–37. John Wiley and Sons.

French, J. and Adams, L. (1986). From analysis to synthesis. Theories of health education. *Health Ed. J.*, **45(2)**, 71–4.

Health Education Authority. (1996). *Sun Know-How Campaign*. Health Education Authority.

Maben, J. and Macleod-Clark, J. (1995). Health promotion: a concept analysis. *J. Adv. Nursing*, **22**, 1158–65.

Macleod-Clark, J. (1993). From sick nursing to health nursing: evolution or revolution? In: *Research in Health Promotion and Nursing* (J. Wilson-Barnett and J. Macleod-Clark, eds), pp. 256–270. Macmillan.

Muir-Gray, J. A. and Fowler, G. (1984). *Essentials of Preventative Medicine*, pp. 45–50. Blackwell Scientific Publications.

Neuman, B. (1989). *The Neuman Systems Model*, 2nd edn. Appleton and Lange.

Norton, D., McLaren, R. and Exton-Smith, A. N. (1975). *An Investigation of Geriatric Nursing Problems in Hospital*. Churchill Livingstone.

Orem, D. (1985). *Nursing: Concepts of Practice*. McGraw Hill.

Prochaska, J. and DiClemente, C. (1984). *The Transtheoretical Approach: Crossing Traditional Foundations of Change*. Don Jones/Irwin.

Roper, N., Logan, W. W. and Tierney, A. J. (1990). *The Elements of Nursing*, 3rd edn. Churchill Livingstone.

Roy, C. (1984). *Introduction to Nursing: An Adaptation Model*, 2nd edn. Prentice Hall.

Temoshok, L., DiClemente, M. S. and Sweet, D. M. *et al.* (1984). Factors related to patient delay in seeking attention for cutaneous malignant melanoma. *Cancer*, **54**, 3048–53.

Thompson, I. E. (1983). Theoretical models of health education. In: *Scottish Health Education Group: In-service Needs of District Nurses, Health Visitors and Midwives*. Edinburgh Health Education Group.

Tones, B. K. (1987). Devising strategies for preventing drug misuse: the role of the health action model. *Health Ed. Res.*, **2**, 305–17.

Further reading

Clarke, A. (1991). Nurses as role models and health educators. *J. Adv. Nursing*, **16**, 1179–84.

Cribb, A. and Dines, A. (eds) (1993). *Health Promotion: Concepts and Practice.* Blackwell Scientific.

Edelman, C. L. and Mandle, C. L. (1990). *Health Promotion: Throughout the Lifespan.* CV Mosby Co.

Ewles, L. and Simnett, J. (1992). *Promoting Health: A Practical Guide.* Scutari Press.

Kaplan, A. (ed.) (1992). *Health Promotion and Chronic Illness: Discovering a New Quality of Health.* World Health Organization Publications, European Series.

Muir-Gray, J. A. and Fowler, G. (1984). *Essentials of Preventative Medicine.* Blackwell Scientific.

Prochaska, J. O. (1990). What causes people to change from unhealthy to health-enhancing behaviour? *Cancer Prev. J.*, **1(1)**, 38–42.

Prochaska, J. and DiClemente, C. (1984). *The Transtheoretical Approach: Crossing Traditional Foundations of Change.* Don Jones/Irwin.

Tones, K., Telford, S. and Robinson, Y. (1990). *Health Education: Effectiveness and Efficiency.* Chapman and Hall.

Webb, P. (1994). *Health Promotion and Patient Education: A Professional Guide.* Chapman and Hall.

Wilson-Barnett, J. and Macleod-Clark, J. (1993). *Research in Health Promotion and Nursing.* Macmillan.

World Health Organization (1986). *Ottawa Charter for Health Promotion.* World Health Organization and Health and Welfare.

Patient support organizations

Useful Address for Support Groups

Acne Support Group
PO Box 230, Hayes
Middlesex UB4 OUT
Reg Charity No. 1026654
Telephone message service: 0181 561 6868
E-mail: alison@the-asg.demon.co.uk
Website: http://www.m2w3.com/acne

British Dermatological Nursing Group (BDNG)
c/o British Association of Dermatologists
19 Fitzroy Square
London W1P 5HQ
Tel: 0207 383 0266; Fax: 0207 388 5263
E-mail: admin@bad.org.uk

CancerBACUP
3 Bath Place, Rivington Street
London EC2A 3JR
Reg Charity No. 1019719
Cancer information service open 9 am–7 pm
Tel: 0207 696 9003; Fax: 0207 696 9002
Counselling service open 9 am–5.30 pm
Tel: 0207 696 9000
Website: http://www.cancerbacup.org.uk

Cancerlink
11-21 Northdown Street,
London N1 9NB
Reg Charity No. 326430
Tel: 0207 833 2818; Fax: 0207 833 4963
Freephone cancer information helpline: 0800 132 905
E-mail: cancerlink@canlink.demon.co.uk

Changing Faces
1 & 2 Junction Mews
Paddington
London W2 1PN
Reg Charity No. 1011222
Tel: 0207 706 4232
Fax: 0207 706 4234
E-mail: info@changingfaces.co.uk

Hairline International
The Alopecia Patients' Society
Lyons Court
1668 High Street, Knowle
West Midlands B93 0LY
Reg Charity No. 1056204
Tel: 01564 775281
Fax: 01584 782270
Please enclose an A4 sae

Herpes Viruses Association (SPHERE) and
Shingles Support Society
41 North Road
London N7 9DP
Reg Charity No. 291657
Tel: 0207 607 9661 (office and Minicom V)
Tel: 0207 609 9061 (helpline – 24 hours access)
Fax number available on request

National Eczema Society
163 Eversholt Street
London NW1 1BU
Reg Charity No. 1009671
A company limited by guarantee, registered
in England No. 2685083
Tel: 0207 388 4097
Fax: 0207 388 5882
Website: http://www.eczema.org

MARC's line (for skin cancer)
Resource Centre
Royal Southants Hospital
Brinton Terrace
Southampton SO9 4PE
Tel: 01722 415 071

Psoriasis Association
Milton House, 7 Milton Street
Northampton NN2 7JG
Reg Charity No. 257414
Tel: 01604 711129
Fax: 01604 792894

Psoriatic Arthropathy Alliance
PO Box 111, St Albans
Hertfordshire AL2 3JQ
Reg Charity No. 1051169
Tel/Fax: 01923 672837
(Telephone support is provided)
E-mail: info@paalliance.org
Website: http://www.paalliance.org

Skin Deep
44 Hartwell Drive
Kempston
Bedfordshire MK43 8UY
Tel: 01234 840013

Tissue Viability Society
Glanville Centre
Salisbury District Hospital
Salisbury SP2 8BJ
Reg Charity No. 1041915
Tel: 01722 3362772, ext 4057
Fax: 01722 325904
E-mail: tvs@dial.pipex.com
Website: http://www.tvs.org.uk

Wound Care Society
PO Box 170
Huntingdon PE18 7PL
Reg Charity No. 1013304
Tel/Fax: 01480 434401

Index